Basic Practices of the
Universal Healing Tao

Basic Practices

of the Universal Healing Tao

An Illustrated Guide to Levels 1 through 6

Mantak Chia
and William U. Wei

Destiny Books
Rochester, Vermont • Toronto, Canada

Destiny Books
One Park Street
Rochester, Vermont 05767
www.destinybooks.com

Destiny Books is a division of Inner Traditions International

Originally published in Thailand in 2008 by Universal Tao Publications under the title *Chi Cards—Book I: Formulas for Immortality*

Library of Congress Cataloging-in-Publication Data
Chia, Mantak, 1944–
 Basic practices of the universal healing Tao : an illustrated guide to levels 1 through 6 / Mantak Chia and William U. Wei.
  p. cm.
 Includes index.
 ISBN 978-1-59477-334-1 (pbk.) — ISBN 978-1-59477-514-7 (e-book)
 1. Qi gong. 2. Tai chi. 3. Exercise. 4. Massage. 5. Mind and body.
I. Wei, William U. II. Title.
 RA781.8.C46918 2012
 613.7'1489—dc23

                                                                                                    2012017265

Printed and bound in the United States by Lake Book Manufacturing, Inc.
The text stock is SFI certified. The Sustainable Forestry Initiative® program promotes sustainable forest management.

10 9 8 7 6 5 4 3 2 1

Text design and layout by Priscilla Baker
This book was typeset in Garamond Premier Pro with Present and Futura used as display typefaces

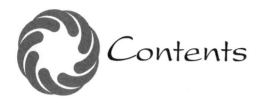 Contents

Preface   vii

Acknowledgments   ix

Putting the First Six Levels of the Universal
Healing Tao System into Practice   xi

Introduction   1

1 ● **LEVEL ONE**   8

    The Inner Smile   16

    Wisdom Chi Kung   20

    The Alchemy of Sexual Energy   24

    Healing Light of the Tao   30

    Chi Self-Massage   34

    The Six Healing Sounds   40

    Iron Shirt Chi Kung   46

    Healing Love through the Tao   58

2 ● **LEVEL TWO**   70

    Bone Marrow Nei Kung   73

    Fusion of Five Elements   98

    The Inner Structure of Tai Chi   113

3 ● LEVEL THREE   132

  Taoist Cosmic Healing   136

  Chi Nei Tsang   152

  Cosmic Fusion   182

  The Healing Energy of Shared Consciousness   202

4 ● LEVEL FOUR   208

  Energy Balance through the Tao   215

  Tan Tien Chi Kung   227

  Simple Chi Kung   236

  Cosmic Detox   242

  Cosmic Astrology   247

  Tendon Nei Kung   249

  Fusion of the Eight Psychic Channels   258

5 ● LEVEL FIVE   270

  Taoist Astral Healing   274

  Advanced Chi Nei Tsang   284

  Golden Elixir Chi Kung   302

  Tai Chi Fa Jin   319

6 ● LEVEL SIX   328

  The Taoist Soul Body   332

  Karsai Nei Tsang   354

  Tai Chi Wu Style   373

About the Authors   385

The Universal Healing Tao System and
Training Center   387

Index   389

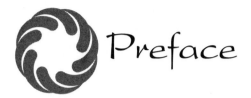 Preface

Many years ago, I discovered the Universal Healing Tao books and a whole new way of approaching life. The books led me to Universal Healing Tao workshops, where I eventually met Master Mantak Chia and began my internal practice in the Universal Healing Tao system.

Over time, I learned that the Universal Healing Tao system consists of many formulas, which have been handed down through the centuries in an instructor-student relationship. As students master these formulas, they gain the opportunity to experience their own self-realization/enlightenment. Like my fellow students, I stumbled for years with trying to follow these formulas from the Universal Healing Tao books. Over time, I worked with Master Chia to develop condensed formulas to assist me in my practice. Instead of fumbling through the many pages of the many books, the condensed formulas allowed me to proceed in my practice much more smoothly.

Those condensed formulas have now been reproduced in this book for the ease of Universal Healing Tao students around the world. The condensed formulas found here were originally the size of playing cards, so they could be easily carried anywhere. Now all six sets of cards have been combined into one book, allowing you to access all of the Universal Healing Tao's basic practices at any time. In book form, the condensed formulas are easier to read and follow. If you find that you need a fuller explanation of any given practice, we have provided page numbers at the beginning of each summarized practice referencing the Universal Healing Tao book where the practice is described in more detail.*

*Note: All reference page numbers refer to the revised editions of these books as published by Destiny Books, Rochester, Vermont. The relevant title in which to locate each reference is indicated by the section heading in the present text.

These condensed formulas provide a unique and practical way of approaching and working with your practice, not only for beginners, but also as a teaching aid for certified instructors and practitioners. The chi formulas presented here will simplify your understanding and practice of the many Universal Healing Tao formulas.

YOUR FRIEND IN THE TAO,

W. U. WEI (*WEI TZU*)

THE PROFESSOR

MASTER OF NOTHINGNESS

THE MYTH THAT TAKES THE MYSTERY OUT OF MYSTICISM

Acknowledgments

The Universal Tao Publications staff involved in the preparation and production of *The Basic Practices of the Universal Healing Tao* extend our gratitude to the many generations of Taoist Masters who have passed on their special lineage, in the form of an unbroken oral transmission, over thousands of years. We thank Taoist Master I Yun (Yi Eng) for his openness in transmitting the formulas of Taoist Inner Alchemy.

We offer our eternal gratitude and love to our parents and teachers for their many gifts to us. Remembering them brings joy and satisfaction to our continued efforts in presenting the Universal Healing Tao system. As always, their contribution has been crucial in presenting the concepts and techniques of the Universal Healing Tao.

We wish to thank the thousands of unknown men and women of the Chinese healing arts who developed many of the methods and ideas presented in this book.

We thank the many contributors essential to this book's final form: the editorial and production staff at Inner Traditions/Destiny Books for their efforts to clarify the text and produce a handsome new edition of the book and Gail Rex for her line edit of the new edition.

We wish to thank the following people for their assistance in producing the earlier editions of this book: Bob Zuraw for sharing his kindness, healing techniques, and Taoist understandings; Matthew Koren for his editorial work and writing contributions, as well as his ideas for the cover; Otto Thamboon for his artisic contributions to the revised edition of this book; our senior instructors, Wilbert Wils and Saumya

x   Acknowledgments

Wils, for their insightful contributions to the revised edition; and special thanks to Charles Morris, without whom the book would not have come to be, for inspiring and reorganizing the book.

A special thanks goes to our Thai production team: Hirunyathorn Punsan, Saysunee Yongyod, Udon Jandee, and Saniem Chaisam.

Putting the First Six Levels of the Universal Healing Tao System into Practice

The practices described in this book have been used successfully for thousands of years by Taoists trained by personal instruction. Readers should not undertake the practice without receiving personal transmission and training from a certified instructor of the Universal Healing Tao, since certain of these practices, if done improperly, may cause injury or result in health problems. This book is intended to supplement individual training by the Universal Healing Tao and to serve as a reference guide for these practices. Anyone who undertakes these practices on the basis of this book alone does so entirely at his or her own risk.

The meditations, practices, and techniques described herein are not intended to be used as an alternative or substitute for professional medical treatment and care. If any readers are suffering from illnesses based on mental or emotional disorders, an appropriate professional health care practitioner or therapist should be consulted. Such problems should be corrected before you start training.

Neither the Universal Healing Tao nor its staff and instructors can be responsible for the consequences of any practice or misuse of the information contained in this book. If the reader undertakes any exercise without strictly following the instructions, notes, and warnings, the responsibility must lie solely with the reader.

This book does not attempt to give any medical diagnosis, treatment, prescription, or remedial recommendation in relation to any human disease, ailment, suffering, or physical condition whatsoever.

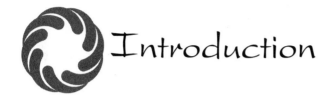 # Introduction

We are dynamically connected to the infinite. "As above, so below" is an echo of wisdom heard from sages and mystics throughout the ages. When we can connect to and absorb the energy that surrounds us, we are able to tap into the many splendors of the universe.

The two main forces that are around and within us are electricity and magnetism, which the Tao refers to collectively as *chi*. (The closest Western term for this life-force energy is *bioelectromagnetism*.) For the past five thousand years, Taoists have utilized this bioelectromagnetic energy to enhance their way of life and establish a relationship with the universe. *Bio* signifies life, *electro* refers to the universal (yang) energies of the stars and planets, and the *magnetic* force refers to the earth (yin) force—gravity—present on all planets and stars. As we align ourselves with these forces, we become a conduit for absorbing and digesting these energies through the body, mind, and spirit, thereby establishing a direct connection with the universe.

Humans normally access bioelectromagnetic energy through food and air. Plants absorb the universal energies of the sun and the magnetic energies of the earth; they digest and transform them, thereby making these energies available to all living beings. Rather than waiting until the energy in the universe has been processed through plants, the Taoist goes directly to the source of this primordial energy. Through the Chinese methods of cultivating energy known as Chi Kung and meditation, the Taoists directly tap into the source of energy all around us and focus it precisely.

Through these internal quests, the ancient Taoists discovered a doorway to the universe: the more we open our internal energy, the more we are capable of connecting to the forces of energy around us. These practices are known as "Inner Alchemy," because they offer us a way to positively influence the changes that naturally happen within us and around us every day.

THE UNIVERSAL HEALING TAO SYSTEM

The Tao is how the river flows, how the sun glows, how the wind blows, how the tree grows, and how a seed becomes a rose. It is in everything that moves or does not move. The only way to understand the Tao is to feel it. The only way to feel it is to practice it, and the only reason to practice the Tao is because it feels good.

The Tao is not a religion; it is a practice of individual self-discovery, so that whoever you are, you can simply become better at it. Taoist practices can teach you how to breathe, sleep, urinate, defecate, sit, stand, walk, and exchange sexual energy in harmony with the natural flow of the universe. Everything starts with a thought, and every thought is a vibration that energetically manifests in our lives and in the universe. The Universal Healing Tao explores these subtle energy vibrations in its diverse practices, which can awaken you to the ways you see, taste, hear, smell, and feel; it will enhance your experience of your life in every moment.

The Universal Healing Tao system is based on ten-thousand-year-old Taoist formulas, and it has continued to evolve over the last fifty-five years in response to Master Chia's research and training. The system is comprised of four Inner Alchemy healing arts, each of which cultivates an aspect of our being: the Living Tao, Chi Nei Tsang, Cosmic Healing, and the Immortal Tao. Each of these arts consists of many different practices that are performed by individuals seeking to refine their relationships to themselves and the universe.

The Living Tao focuses on the emotional body and can be practiced in our normal living environments within our families, businesses, and religious affiliations. It enhances our perceptions, body awareness, and daily experiences. Chi Nei Tsang explores the physical body. It is a hands-on healing practice that you can perform on yourself as well as others. Cosmic

Healing, which is devoted to the refinement of the energy body, works to heal the self and others via direct contact with the universal healing energies that we know as the heavenly, earthly, and atmospheric forces.

The Immortal Tao focuses on the spirit body and is the highest form of Inner Alchemy. To be truly successful with its practices, you need to be isolated and totally detached from all earthly connections. For this reason, it is usually practiced by people in the later stages of their lives, when immediate family, friends, and occupations are no longer a central focus.

All of the practices in the Universal Healing Tao system cultivate our ability to work with internal and external energy. The word in the Tao for energy is *chi,* thus the chi formulas are energy formulas. Through them, you will become aware of your own energy and the energy around you. After discovering your energy, you can use these formulas to help purify, transform, regenerate, and transcend it, further discovering your relationship to the energy surrounding you.

The Universal Healing Tao system offers five stages for mastering chi.

1. **Conserving chi.** In the Universal Tao system, our first goal is to learn to conserve our chi; when a battery is totally drained, it is harder to charge. Conservation of chi will help us gain more chi. To have more chi we first need to maintain control of the gates through which energy normally leaks out and constantly drains our life force. Without knowing how to conserve the chi that we already have, what is the point of acquiring more?

   We leak energy in the following ways:
   - Through our reproductive system
   - Through negative emotion
   - Through constantly turning our senses outward
   - Through poor diet and eating habits
   - Through improper or shallow breathing

2. **Balancing chi.** Learning to balance chi is the second step to keeping a smooth and harmonious flow of energy moving throughout the whole body. If our energy is imbalanced, we may have too much energy in some places and not enough in others; we may also be too

yang or too yin. We may have an excess or deficiency of heat, cold, damp, or dryness. This imbalanced energy tends to make us go to extremes.

3. **Transforming chi.** Transforming chi is the third phase and allows practitioners access to more beneficial energies. For example, through the Sexual Chi Kung practices taught in the Universal Tao (the course known as Healing Love through the Tao), we can transform sexual energy back into basic life-force chi. Through other practices (such as the Inner Smile, the Six Healing Sounds, and Fusion of the Five Elements) we learn to transform negative emotional chi into positive virtuous chi. Thus chi is not only the foundation of our health; it is also the basis of spiritual development in the Tao.

4. **Increasing chi.** Once we have accomplished the three previous phases of mastering chi, we then learn to increase it. Chi pervades all of heaven and earth. In Cosmic Healing Chi Kung we learn time-tested ways to tap into these unlimited and transpersonal reservoirs of chi and greatly expand the amount of energy available to us. It is very important to first master the stages of conservation, balance, and transformation before we emphasize increasing our chi. Otherwise we may waste the energy we bring in, or we may inadvertently amplify the imbalanced or negative energies that we have not yet learned to bring under control.

5. **Expanding chi.** Finally, we learn to extend our mind to tap in to the vast chi of the universe to heal our body, mind, and spirit and to heal other people. The Universal Healing Tao practices sensitize your hands and body to the feeling and movement of chi. You can learn to use your mind/eye/heart power (Yi) to absorb Cosmic Chi and multiply it in your body, then send it to restore balance in others.

As you practice, you will discover that the formulas are interconnected—from the initial practice (Inner Smile) all the way to the last one (Reunion of Heaven and Man). No matter how far you get with the system you will feel better, look better, understand more, and live longer. Furthermore, you will energetically carry everything you discover through your practices beyond this life.

THE LEVELS OF PRACTICE INCLUDED IN THIS BOOK

This book is broken down into six levels as follows:

Level One includes the foundational practices of the Universal Healing Tao, including the Inner Smile, the Six Healing Sounds, the Microcosmic Orbit, Iron Shirt Chi Kung, and Chi Self-Massage, among others. These are basic, beginner-level practices that provide a safe and thorough introduction to Universal Healing Tao concepts and forms.

Level Two takes practitioners a little bit deeper into the Chi Kung and Tai Chi Chi Kung forms. It also offers the first series of Inner Alchemy exercises—the Fusion of the Five Elements.

Level Three provides an introduction to the Cosmic Healing practices, teaching ways of cultivating the heaven and earth forces within the body. It also offers the first set of practices dedicated to the healing of the physical body—Chi Nei Tsang.

Level Four takes the practitioner deeper into the body, growing tendons and developing the lower tan tien with Empty Force. It also provides guidelines for daily living with Simple Chi Kung and Cosmic Detox.

Level Five presents a deeper exploration of Cosmic Healing, Advanced Chi Nei Tsang, and Golden Elixir Chi Kung, as well as the discharge power of Tai Chi. These practices begin to cultivate the refined energies that are a vital step on the road to immortality.

Level Six offers formulas at the higher levels of Cosmic Healing, Chi Nei Tsang, and Tai Chi Chi Kung. These advanced practices develop and strengthen the energy body, providing glimpses of the ageless and timeless Way.

THE COMPLETE UNIVERSAL
HEALING TAO SYSTEM

This volume offers the basic Universal Healing Tao practices, which constitute just the first half of the Universal Healing Tao system. By 2020 the written system should be complete, with the publication of another twenty-one books on topics such as cosmic astrology, Greater Kan and Li practices, and Christ's teachings within the Tao. This next series of books will delineate another six levels of practice, moving completely into the Immortal Tao.

Together, the twelve levels will encompass the entire Universal Healing Tao system—more than five hundred formulas—completing the roadmap to immortality. Becoming immortal is a whole process, akin to building a house or a temple (your body) for doing practices. You must begin with a solid foundation (the basic formulas), then add the wiring, plumbing, insulation, rooms, floors, siding, and roof (the different levels within the healing arts). Ultimately, you learn to transform this temple into a space ship (through the Immortal Tao practices), which can take you beyond the North Star into your own immortality.

This complete roadmap has never before appeared in any single written work because bringing all of the material together is simply an enormous undertaking. For centuries, the teachings of the Tao were passed down via the spoken word, from the mountain sages to students who were willing to venture into the remotest areas without any provisions or support, and who often took years to find their masters. It has already taken more than thirty years to complete this first section of the system in writing—and more than sixty years of research, conceptualization, cultivation, systemization, instruction, and practice. This project has only been possible because of the dedication, enthusiasm, and perseverance of Master Chia for the Tao and for his master; and because of my gratitude for Master Chia and the Tao. Together, we are determined to complete the task for all of humankind, so that all may have the opportunity for their own self-realization (enlightenment and immortality). We all need to achieve this realization to complete humanity's transformation into our true divine being.

The Tao teaches us not only how to plant (root) and grow our seed (energy or essence) into a tree but also how to sexually cultivate the seed to bear fruit, without losing our original essence. Our tree (cultivated energy) will bear fruit by the hundreds, so we will have an abundance to share with others who are sincere and deserving. Now think: how many seeds are there to share within each piece of fruit that we bear? If we cultivate our original seed in the Tao, we can share thousands of seeds for the good of others and never lose our original essence: this is what you can accomplish when you practice the formulas of the Universal Healing Tao on a daily basis.

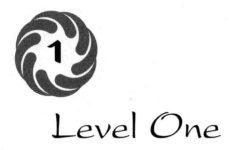

Level One

Level One comprises the most basic practices of the Universal Healing Tao system. In this level there are thirty formulas, which have been described in great detail in the following Universal Healing Tao books from Destiny Books: *The Inner Smile, The Six Healing Sounds, Chi Self-Massage, Healing Light of the Tao, The Alchemy of Sexual Energy, Wisdom Chi Kung, Iron Shirt Chi Kung,* and *Healing Love Through the Tao.* You can refer to these books for more details about any of the practices presented here.

THE GOALS OF THE LEVEL ONE PRACTICES

The broad goals of these practices include learning to feel your energy, transforming negative energy into positive energy, recycling sexual energy, and training your body to be a strong container for energy.

Feeling Your Energy

Before you can cultivate your energy, you need to become aware of it. All of the Healing Tao practices, beginning with the Inner Smile, help you focus your awareness on the many subtle expressions of energy within you.

Transforming Negative Energy into Positive Energy

Negative emotions are normal. Feelings such as impatience, anger, and worry happen every day. We call such feelings "negative" because when they stay in us too long they become stagnant and detrimental to our health. Western doctors now realize that a lot of sickness is caused by negative emotions: anger increases blood pressure and puts stress on the heart. This is contrary to what happens with positive emotions like love, joy, generosity, happiness, and trust, which nurture us.

We can learn how to change the negative into positive energy to improve our health and spiritual energy. What the Taoists discovered is that negative energy can be used to cultivate positive energy. Changing the negative into positive, such as changing anger into happiness, is also known in Taoism and alchemy as "changing lead into gold." This is not only beneficial to the practitioner but also to everyone around: when our loved ones are sad, angry, or depressed, we can send love and gentleness to them and make them feel better.

Recycling Sexual Energy

In Taoist thought sexual energy or *ching* is the source of all life and creativity. It is the basic resource, which can be transformed first into chi (life-force energy) and then into shen (spiritual energy). When we feel sexual arousal and desire, the sexual hormones are activated. This is the beginning of the inner alchemy of sexual energy. In the Taoist Healing Love practices this energy is recycled and used to regenerate the body's internal energy.

Cultivating a Strong Container

Our bodies are like wiring that must be strong enough to carry the electric charge placed on them. In other words, we must develop and strengthen our bodies so that they can contain the powerful chi that we cultivate in our practices. The Tai Chi Chi Kung practice and the Chi Nei Tsang practices are vital for developing the physical body's strength and sensitivity.

THE INNER SMILE

Theory: The first step in this Inner Alchemy process is to feel the internal energy. The only way to cultivate the Tao is to feel it inside yourself. Through the Inner Smile formula you communicate mentally with your five vital organs and their yang counterparts, using your eyes to smile down along lines that connect with each part of your body. Doing this on a daily basis will help you develop a personal relationship with yourself on physical, emotional, mental, and spiritual levels.

Concept: Smiling energy is generated by your heart when you focus your eyes into it with positive thoughts. This initiates a parasympathetic response in your autonomic nervous system, creating feelings of relaxation and love in your body. When you move that smile down through your body, it will respond with positive loving energy. This is how we learn to generate love within ourselves instead of taking it from others; furthermore, an abundance of such love within us will spread to others energetically—without our trying to "give it" away to anyone.

Purpose: When you greet someone with a warm hug or a smile that person tends to respond in kind; your internal body parts will do the same. Directing loving energy to your organs will leave you feeling relaxed, calm, and at peace. This creates the proper internal environment for taking the next step in cultivating your internal energy. For this reason, the Inner Smile should always be the first step in your daily practice and a preliminary to every other formula.

THE SIX HEALING SOUNDS

Theory: When you work with internal energy you create heat, so the second step in your Inner Alchemy practice is to learn how to cool the energy down. The Six Healing Sounds practice effectively cools the energy in your organs. So you start your daily practice with the Inner Smile and end it with the Six Healing Sounds. Once you learn these first two formulas you can safely add the next 240+ formulas of the Universal Healing Tao system in between them.

Concept: The connective tissue (fascia) around your vital organs absorbs excess heat and releases it through your skin and digestive tract. When you urinate, defecate, yawn, belch, or sweat, you release heat; these everyday body functions are a part of your cooling system. If years of improper diet and lack of exercise have impaired the body's ability to release excess heat, the vital organs can malfunction or break down altogether. If you are driving your car down the highway and your dashboard temperature light goes on, you know the engine is overheating. If you do not stop the car and cool the engine down it can cease to function—just like your organs.

Purpose: The Six Healing Sounds formula activates your cooling system on a daily basis. Its postures restructure the connective tissue around your vital organs so that they function properly, and the individual sounds release condensed heat. Practicing this formula before bedtime every night is an effective way to release the cares and worries (condensed heat) of the day.

WISDOM CHI KUNG

Theory: In this practice we move vital organ energy to specific sections of the brain, then send it out to the universe. In the emptiness of the universe we multiply this energy and draw it back into the brain. This practice charges the brain, increasing its thinking power and wisdom by opening it up to universal consciousness.

Concept: When the universe was created eons ago, our collective consciousness manifested a thought and sent it out into the emptiness of the cosmos. Our thought hit the emptiness and multiplied, forming the universe (Big Bang theory)—just as our reflection comes back to us when we look into a mirror. This is how everything is created: by forming a thought and sending it out into the emptiness. We create manufacturing blueprints with our thoughts all the time, but we are not conscious of doing so. Becoming aware of this process helps us to create thoughts and manifestations that are beneficial to all.

Purpose: These formulas teach you to expand your consciousness by expanding your brain energetically into the universe. This process exercises and strengthens your brain's thinking capacity, helping you generate true wisdom.

THE ALCHEMY OF SEXUAL ENERGY

Theory: To further expand your consciousness you can activate the three fires (tan tien, kidney, and heart) into the three tan tiens (upper/crown mind, middle/heart mind, and lower/tan tien mind) through the Microcosmic Orbit. This is moving the three minds into one, which gives you Yi power. Once this transition has been completed, you can open your awareness to the cosmos, moving fortified energy in the six directions (up and down, left and right, front and back). This will give you a feeling of buoyancy supported by the six directions and the experience of being the center of the universe.

Concept: We will learn how to harness excess sexual energy and transform it into chi. When we circulate sexual energy in the Microcosmic Orbit, we transform it into self-healing energy that can be stored in the organs and the three tan tiens. In learning to open the three tan tiens to the six directions, the Taoist practitioner combines mind power with the extension of chi to draw cosmic energy into the body. When we learn to flow in this way with the energy of the Tao, life ceases to be a struggle.

Purpose: This practice is a continuation of the Microcosmic Orbit, activating the sexual energy for additional strength then moving this creative energy through the orbit while extending it down through the legs. Using the six direction formula by activating the three tan tiens and fires allows you to connect with the cosmos and further expand your awareness.

HEALING LIGHT OF THE TAO

Theory: With this formula you can reconnect to your physical beginning and become aware of the internal energy moving in your body. When each of us was growing in our mother's womb, our connection to her—

to life itself—was the umbilical cord that linked her body to our navel: from this sacred energy we formed our bodies. The energy moved from the navel down to the sacrum, then up the spine to the crown (Governor Channel), then down the front of the body (Functional Channel), back to the navel. This is the Microcosmic Orbit, and as long as you are alive your energy still moves within it, though you may not be conscious of it. Once you become aware of this flowing energy (light), you can use it to heal any internal energy blockage in your body.

Concept: We can become conscious of this movement by tracing it with our mind's eye. Taking in small sips of air to help focus the mind on the moving energy, we can trace the Microcosmic Orbit through fourteen points up the spine and down the front of the body. Then we connect each point on the spine to its counter point (Ming Men to Navel, Sacrum to Sexual Palace, Crown point to perineum, T11 to sternum, Wing point to Heart Center, C7 to Throat Center, and Jade Pillow to Mid-Eyebrow), spreading energy across the body and healing ourselves section by section.

Purpose: After we learn how to feel the internal smiling energy (Inner Smile), cool it down (Six Healing Sounds), and break up any blockages (Chi Self-Massage), we practice the Microcosmic Orbit meditation to direct our light energy to heal the body. This is how we learn to move the love that we generated, which will ultimately spread to others across time and space.

CHI SELF-MASSAGE

Theory: Your body is a series of energy rivers that travel from your vital organs throughout your body to the surface of your skin. These rivers are the meridians, acupuncture points, channels, and nerve endings that are the communications network of your body—like the electrical wiring in your house. The paths can become blocked from inside the organs or within the networking itself, resulting in miscommunication and malfunction.

Concept: By simply touching the extremities (skin) of your body, you can connect daily to your vital organs and open up any blockages within the networking. When you massage your face, neck, chest, hands, arms, legs, and feet you release stress and tension from the whole system.

Purpose: Living in our unnatural environments puts a lot of stress on our bodies—from supposedly "simple" activities like driving a car to complex financial responsibilities, overexposure to light and sound, improper diet, unfit sleeping conditions, and lack of exercise. We all need a simple technique for releasing built-up stress and the blockages it can cause. By applying Chi Self-Massage formulas after daily practice (and any long sitting or standing period), or any time you feel tension throughout the day, you can literally keep in touch with yourself, opening the body and the vital organs as needed.

IRON SHIRT CHI KUNG

Theory: With correct structural body alignment you can root yourself into the earth, creating an energetic grounding effect similar to the grounding wire of an electrical outlet. Proper grounding ensures that any excess energy you generate during your Inner Alchemy practices will automatically release itself from your body and aura. The seven standing Iron Shirt postures included in this book (Embracing the Tree, Holding the Golden Urn, Golden Turtle Immersing in Water, Water Buffalo Emerging from Water, Golden Phoenix Washes Its Feathers, Iron Bridge, and Iron Bar) should be practiced daily.

Concept: These postures, when practiced with the Iron Shirt packing technique, will build an Iron Shirt body to protect your vital organs. Like packing an egg in an air-filled balloon, then surrounding it in further layers of air-filled balloons, the Iron Shirt practices put protection in the right places. The egg is our vital organs, the air is the chi pressure that we create through small inhalations, and the balloons are the connective tissue (fascia) that surrounds the vital organs.

Purpose: By simply standing and packing in the Iron Shirt postures for five to ten minutes a day, you will root yourself to earth and build a strong body that can live for hundreds of years. When you are rooted no one can push you around physically, mentally, emotionally, or spiritually, because they are pushing the earth, not you—and no one can push the earth around. Why do you need to live a hundred years or more? To do all of the Universal Healing Tao Inner Alchemy practices for your transformation.

HEALING LOVE THROUGH THE TAO

Theory: What is chicken soup? You boil a chicken in a pot of water for a few hours, then take the chicken out. Which would you rather eat, the chicken or the broth? The broth is what you would eat, because the broth has all the essence of the chicken in it: it has flavor and nuance and energy, while the chicken itself would taste like nothing at this point. Try it.

The Healing Love practices similarly "cook" the vital essence in your genitals and draw it up your spine into your brain. This allows for a total body orgasm without the loss of your sexual fluids (semen and hormones), which your body can then use as needed to create and nourish your cells. These same formulas apply to women for the loss of sexual fluids during their menstrual cycle.

Concept: You have the ability to completely experience your sexual energy and take it to new highs without losing any of your vital creative energy. The Universal Healing Tao Healing Love practices help you to build your vital energies and use them to heal yourself and your loved one. Through these practices you will learn to manage your sexual energy instead of being controlled by it.

Purpose: Single Cultivation practices help you slow down the sexual energy so that you can begin to manage it. These practices include Ovarian Breathing, Ovarian Compression, and the Egg Exercise. Dual Cultivation practices—like the Orgasmic Upward Draw and the Valley Orgasm—teach you to work together with your partner to heal yourselves and flow together in a harmonious, monogamous, long-lasting relationship.

THE INNER SMILE

Front Line: The Functional Channel

(Pages 36–41)

1. Be aware of smiling cosmic energy in front of you and breathe it into your eyes.
2. Allow smiling energy to enter the point between your eyebrows. Let it flow into your nose and cheeks, and let it lift up the corners of your mouth, bringing your tongue to rest on your palate.
3. Smile down to your neck, throat, thyroid, parathyroid, and thymus.
4. Smile into your heart, feeling joy and love spread out from there to the lungs, liver, spleen, pancreas, kidneys, and genitals.

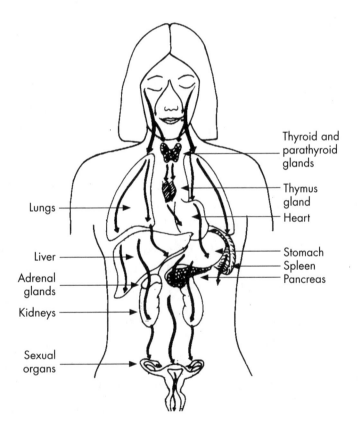

Front line smile:
major vital organs

⊙ Middle Line: The Digestive Tract
(Pages 41–43)

1. Bring smiling energy into the eyes, then down to the mouth.
2. Swallow saliva as you smile down to your stomach, small intestine (duodenum, jejunum, and ileum), large intestine (ascending colon, transverse colon, and descending colon), rectum, and anus.

⊙ Back Line: The Governor Channel
(Pages 43–47)

1. Smile, and look upward about 3 inches into your mid-eyebrow point and pituitary gland.
2. Direct your smile to the Third Room, the small cavity deep in the center of your brain. Feel the room expand and grow with the bright golden light shining through the brain.

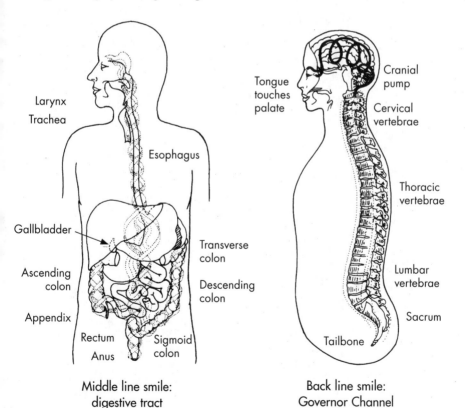

Middle line smile:
digestive tract

Back line smile:
Governor Channel

3. Smile into the thalamus, pineal gland (Crystal Room), and the left and right sides of the brain.

4. Smile to the midbrain and the brain stem, then to the base of your skull.

5. Smile down to the seven cervical vertebrae, the twelve thoracic vertebrae, the five lumbar vertebrae, then the sacrum and the tailbone.

6. Refresh the loving, soothing smile energy in your eyes, then smile down the front, middle, and back lines in succession. Now do all of them at once, feeling bathed in a cooling waterfall or glowing sunshine of cosmic energy, smiles, joy, and love.

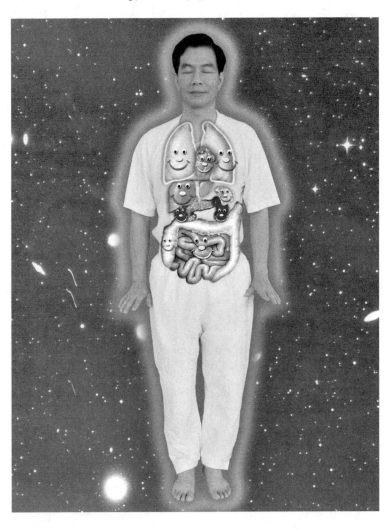

❂ Collect Energy in Navel

(Pages 47–48)

1. Gather all the smiling energy in your navel area—about 1.5 inches inside your body. Spiral that energy with your mind or your hands from the center point to the outside. (Don't go above diaphragm or below pubic bone.)

2. Men spiral clockwise 36 times, then counterclockwise 24 times, returning energy toward the center. Women spiral out counterclockwise 36 times, then inward clockwise 24 times. Finish by storing energy safely in the navel.

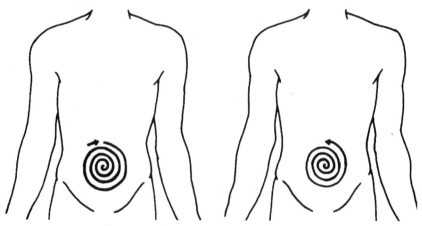

Collecting smiling energy in the navel for men

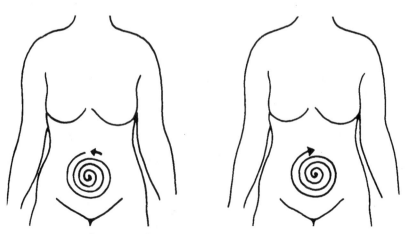

Collecting smiling energy in the navel for women

WISDOM CHI KUNG

🌀 Spinal Cord Breathing

(Pages 60–61)

This exercise will activate the cranial and sacral pumps and loosen the joints of the spine.

1. Stand comfortably with your feet hip-width apart and your elbows and knees slightly bent.
2. Inhale and expand your chest. As you exhale, bend your upper back forward and pull your chin toward your chest. At the same time, tuck your tailbone under you and round your back by bringing your elbows toward one another in front of your chest.
3. Smile, inhale again, expand the chest, tuck your chin toward your throat, and raise your crown. Bring your arms out toward your sides.
4. Repeat steps 2 and 3 thirty-six times.

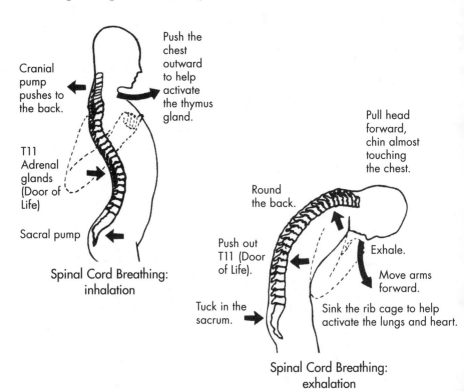

Cranial pump pushes to the back.

Push the chest outward to help activate the thymus gland.

T11 Adrenal glands (Door of Life)

Sacral pump

Spinal Cord Breathing: inhalation

Pull head forward, chin almost touching the chest.

Round the back.

Push out T11 (Door of Life).

Exhale.

Move arms forward.

Tuck in the sacrum.

Sink the rib cage to help activate the lungs and heart.

Spinal Cord Breathing: exhalation

⟳ Wisdom Chi Kung Summary Practice
(Pages 128–33)

1. Smile down, emptying your mind and filling the abdominal brain with chi.
2. Activate the tan tien fire and kidney fire, retaining your awareness at the tan tien. Draw in cosmic energy, not your own.
3. Activate heart fire (Imperial Fire) creating softness and joy.
4. Smile down and empty your mind into the kidneys, as blue Kidney Chi rises and fills the back part of the brain. Then smile down and empty your mind into the bladder and the sexual organs, whose transformed energy will rise up and fill the center part of the brain.
5. Smile down and empty the mind into the liver and gallbladder. Chi transformed here will rise up and fill the center of the right brain. Smile down into the heart and small intestine, whose chi will fill the front part of the center of the brain. Empty mind into the spleen, stomach,

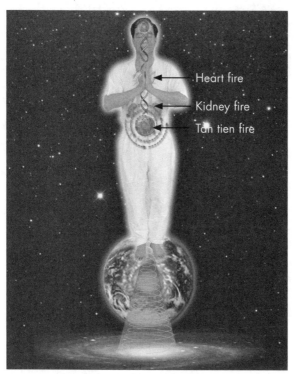

Activation of the three fires: tan tien, kidney, and heart

and pancreas, whose energy will fill the left brain, and then the lungs and large intestine whose energy will fill the front part of the brain.

6. When your mind is empty, it can be filled with transformed energy from all the organs. When your brain is filled with Rainbow Chi, connect with the star of light above you while retaining your awareness at the tan tien.

7. Smile and completely empty your brain to the stars and galaxies. Relax and be completely empty.

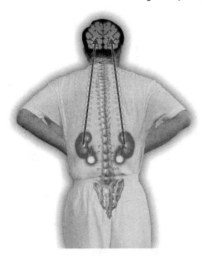

Kidney chi fills both sides of the back of the brain.

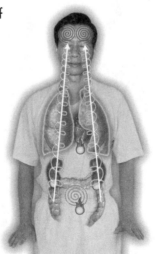

Connect with the star of light above.

Transformed chi from the lungs and large intestines fills the front of the brain.

8. Open yourself with good intentions to universal energies, combining them with the transformed chi at the tan tien. Energy will return to you multiplied to fill the brain and body with wisdom. Empty your brain to the universe again, then fill the mind with higher life force and universal understanding.

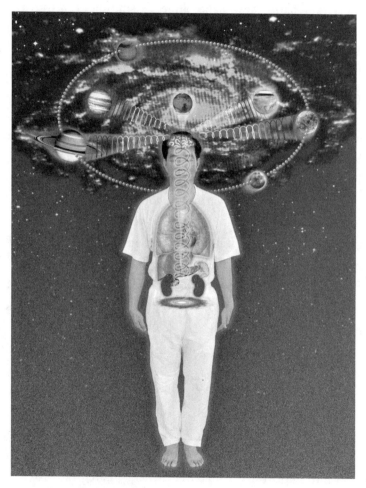

Wisdom Chi Kung fills the whole brain and body with energy transformed by universal understanding.

THE ALCHEMY OF SEXUAL ENERGY

🌀 Activating the Six Directions and the Three Fires

(Pages 131–40)

1. **Below:** Stand with feet together and hands parallel to the ground. Press your hands down and smile, expanding deep into the earth. Push your hands forward and pull them back, drawing chi into the tan tien. Push and pull 3–9 times.

2. **Front:** Become aware of a big fireball in front of you. Scoop it up with your hands and use it to light the fire in your lower tan tien.

3. **Behind:** Expand awareness to the universe behind you. Extend your hands to the back, scoop up the fire, and use it to activate your kidney fire.

4. **Sides:** Raise your hands under your armpits and hold two fireballs. Extend your fingers into your heart. Be aware of infinite space on either side, and feel the warmth of your heart fire.

5. Join your hands together in front of your heart. Connect the heart fire to the kidney fire, kidney fire to the tan tien fire, and the tan tien fire to the heart fire. Circulate as one large triangular fire.

6. Extend your arms in front of you with palms toward your face and the middle fingers extended toward your third eye. Picture a crack at the mid-eyebrow point opening up to let heavenly light shine into the brain and reflect onto the organs. Open and close the third eye 3–9 times.

🌸 Push/Pull Master Practice

7. **Front:** With arms extended forward and palms vertical, push from the scapulae, touching the universe and Cosmic Chi. Pulling in from the scapulae, draw the Universal Chi into your tan tien. Push very far away into the universe, and pull the energy in. Repeat 100–200 times.

8. **Left and right:** Push your hands out to both sides, smiling and touching the universe, then draw the energy into your tan tien. Repeat 3–6 times.

9. **Above:** Extend your arms with palms up and fill the bones with chi. Scoop up the chi and pour it over your crown, touching the crown with your fingertips. Project the chi down to the perineum and into

the earth. Feel the chi spiraling in your tan tien, heart, crown, and in the universe. Continue to gather the energy in from earth, from the universe (at the crown), and bring it into your mid-eyebrow point, then down to the tan tien.

10. Touch your navel and feel the chi spiral faster and faster. Feel your tan tien and the universe spiraling at a fast speed.

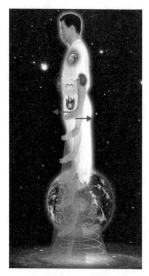

Direction below

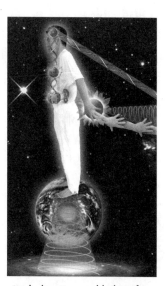

Back direction and kidney fire

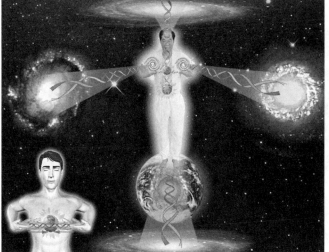

Activate the heart fire.

Activating the six directions and the three fires

THE ALCHEMY OF SEXUAL ENERGY

The Cosmic Orbit Meditation

(Pages 153–84)

Opening the Upper Tan Tien

1. Raise your hands to the universe and pack the bones with chi. Let the North Star and Big Dipper descend into your hands. Pour violet heavenly light from the universe into your crown. Guide this healing light into your brain, down the spine, and deep into your bones, then down to the soles of your feet to connect with the earth at Kidney 1.

2. Touch the back crown point and pour chi into it. Feel chi penetrating to the coccyx. Spiral energy at the heart and crown, and feel the universe spiraling in the six directions, charging the tan tiens.

3. Let any sick energy and negative forces leave the body and go into the earth to be recycled. Extend chi from the universe above down through your body and through the earth to the universe below.

4. Repeat steps 2 and 3 at the mid-crown point, connecting to the perineum.

5. Scoop energy from above and place your fingers on the mid-eyebrow

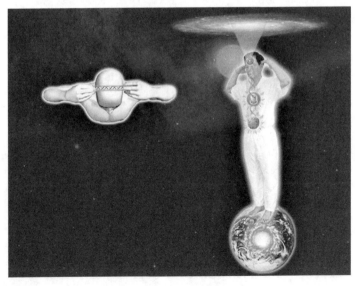

Cutting open the top of the skull

point, letting the chi penetrate to the Jade Pillow at the base of your skull. Then move your fingertips to your upper lip, letting the energy charge your upper palate.

6. Move your fingers to the tops of your ears where—like lasers—they "cut open" the skull and allow chi to bathe the whole brain. Spiral your lower tan tien, heart, and crown, and feel the universe spiraling in all six directions. Gather the chi in your lower tan tien.

7. Move your fingers to the back of the skull, "cutting" as you go; feel energy like a laser beam from the base of your skull to the mid-eyebrow and out to the universe beyond. "Cut" all the way around to the mid-eyebrow point, then touch your upper lips and feel them connect to the tongue and upper palate.

8. Touch the throat center and feel the energy connection to C7. This will activate the thymus, thyroid, and parathyroid glands.

Opening the Middle Tan Tien

9. Recharge from the universe and pour chi over the crown. Touch the heart center and reach through to T5/T6, then out to the universe behind you. Penetrate into the thymus gland, and also into the bones and marrow.

10. Move your hands under your armpits to cut open the middle tan tien. Continue to move your hands around to T5/T6, and beam energy from back to front, and to the universe in front of you. Bring your hands back to the front, cutting as you go.

11. Touch the solar plexus and connect to T11. Feel the sun radiating from T11 through the whole body.

Opening the Lower Tan Tien

12. Recharge with chi and move your hands to your navel, connecting through to the Door of Life and the universe behind you. Cut from the navel around the sides to the Door of Life. Feel your tan tien and the universe spiraling. As you touch the Door of Life, beam energy through to the navel and to the universe in front of you. Move your hands back to the navel, cutting as you go.

13. Move your hands to the pubic bone/sexual center and connect to the sacrum, then touch the sacrum and connect to the sexual center.

🌀 Opening the Bones, Sacrum, and Governing Vessel

14. Touch your hip bones, penetrating deep into the marrow, and laugh inwardly. Move your hands down your legs, squatting as you go, to sink the energy into the ground and the universe below.

15. Touch your heels, raise your sacrum, and wiggle your tailbone to open the area. Squat and send your energy down again, then touch your heels and raise your sacrum again. Squat for a third time, gathering chi from the earth below, and slowly rise up. Touch your coccyx and feel the energy rising up your spine to the crown.

16. Touch the sacrum, feel it expand, and breathe through its 8 holes.

17. Touch the points along the back in turn, and connect each to its energy center on the front: Door of Life to the navel; T11 to the solar plexus; T5 to the heart center; C7 to the throat center; Jade Pillow to the mid-eyebrow point. Feel your tan tien and the universe spiraling at each energy center.

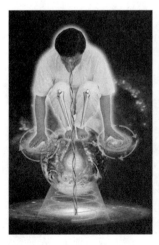

Send chi into the earth and the universe below.

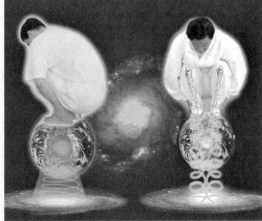

Touch your heels as you begin to rise up.

18. Touch the crown, and feel energy penetrate to the perineum.

19. Continue gathering energy and moving it through the orbit, then touch the navel and bring all the energy into the lower tan tien. Feel it spiraling faster and faster, and the universe spiraling faster and faster, as you maintain inner stillness.

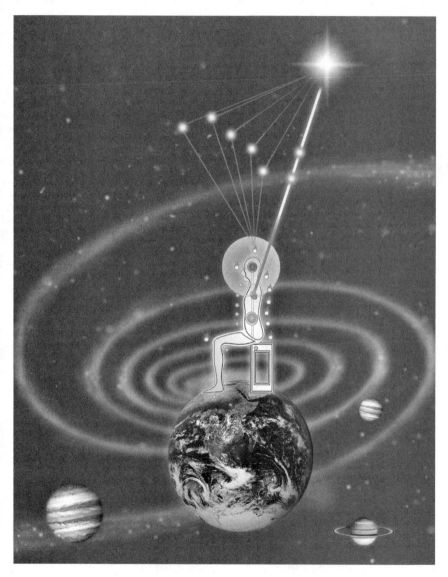

Moving energy through the Cosmic Orbit

HEALING LIGHT OF THE TAO

☯ Opening the Microcosmic Orbit

(Pages 239–56)

Sit comfortably on the sitz bones, with your back straight and chin tucked in slightly. The nine points of the feet should be on the floor, with the shoulders relaxed and the scapulae rounded.

1. Place your right hand on the navel center and the left hand on the pubic bone/sexual center. Send energy from the right hand to the left, then spiral energy at the sexual center with your mind and eyes: 36 times counterclockwise, then 36 times clockwise. Inhale and exhale into the sexual center 9–18 times, feeling chi accumulate.

2. Move your left hand to the perineum, feeling energy radiate down from the navel and sexual center. Spiral energy with mind/eye power at the perineum 36 times counterclockwise then 36 times clockwise, then inhale and exhale into the perineum 9–18 times.

3. Gather energy into a chi ball at the lower tan tien and rotate it top to front to bottom to back, then bring the chi ball into the perineum.

4. Place your left hand on your sacrum and coccyx, right hand on the sexual center. Pull up lightly on the perineum and anus, drawing energy up from the right hand to the left. Spiral this energy at the sacrum and coccyx 36 times in each direction, then inhale and exhale into the area 3–9 times.

5. Move your left hand to the Door of Life and let chi radiate to that point. Spiral a chi ball there 36 times in each direction, then inhale and exhale into the Door of Life 9–18 times.

6. Place your right hand on your sacrum and use your left hand to add the following points to the orbit: T11, the wing point between T5 and T6 (opposite the heart), then the C7 point, Jade Pillow, back of the crown, top of the crown, and the mid-eyebrow point. Spiral a chi ball at each point 36 times in each direction, then inhale and exhale into the point 3–9 times.

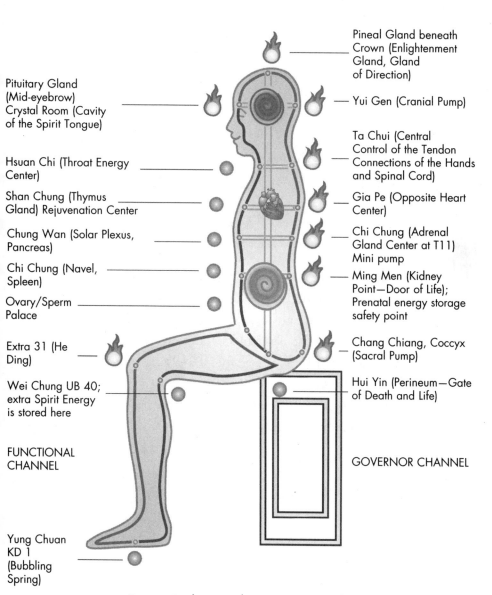

Pineal Gland beneath Crown (Enlightenment Gland, Gland of Direction)

Pituitary Gland (Mid-eyebrow) Crystal Room (Cavity of the Spirit Tongue)

Yui Gen (Cranial Pump)

Hsuan Chi (Throat Energy Center)

Ta Chui (Central Control of the Tendon Connections of the Hands and Spinal Cord)

Shan Chung (Thymus Gland) Rejuvenation Center

Gia Pe (Opposite Heart Center)

Chung Wan (Solar Plexus, Pancreas)

Chi Chung (Adrenal Gland Center at T11) Mini pump

Chi Chung (Navel, Spleen)

Ming Men (Kidney Point—Door of Life); Prenatal energy storage safety point

Ovary/Sperm Palace

Extra 31 (He Ding)

Chang Chiang, Coccyx (Sacral Pump)

Wei Chung UB 40; extra Spirit Energy is stored here

Hui Yin (Perineum—Gate of Death and Life)

FUNCTIONAL CHANNEL

GOVERNOR CHANNEL

Yung Chuan KD 1 (Bubbling Spring)

Energy circulating in the Microcosmic Orbit

7. Press the tip of your tongue against your palate then release it, repeating 9–18 times. Knock your teeth together 18–36 times, then lightly clench and release them. Rotate a chi ball at the palate 36 times each way, then inhale and exhale into the palate 3–9 times.

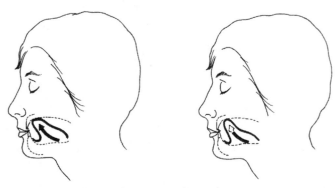

Press the tongue, then release it.

8. Use your left hand to add the throat center, heart center, and solar plexus center: collect energy at each point and spiral it 36 times in each direction, then inhale and exhale into the point.

9. Return energy to the navel and spiral it 36 times in each direction. Inhale and exhale into the navel point 3–9 times, feeling energy pulsing behind the navel.

10. Continue to guide the energy flow through the Microcosmic Orbit as many times as you like, then relax and let the energy flow how-

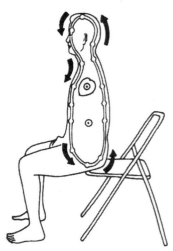

Guide the energy flow through
the Microcosmic Orbit.

ever it wants to. Spend 5–10 minutes at this stage, just feeling your body dissolve into your Original Chi, resting in a state of emptiness.

11. Collect all the energy at your navel and in front of the kidneys. Spiral the energy around the navel 36 times outward and 24 times inward. Men rotate clockwise outward and counterclockwise inward, women the opposite.

12. Rest and finish with Chi Self-Massage.

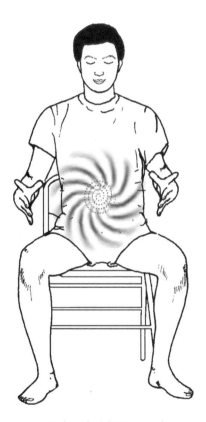

Gather the chi into and around the navel.

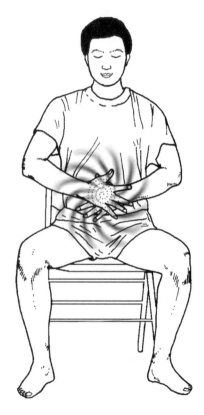

Collect energy at the navel.

CHI SELF-MASSAGE

⟳ Eyes

(Pages 33–40)

1. Rub your hands briskly together as you contract your anus. Place palms on eyes to fill them with energy.
2. Close eyes. Use your fingertips to gently massage the eyeballs through the lids. Massage 6–9 times clockwise, then 6–9 times counterclockwise. Massage around the lids the same number of times.
3. Gently pinch your eyelids between your thumbs and forefingers and pull them outward 6–9 times.
4. With your hands in loose fists, use the lower part of your index fingers to rub the upper and lower bones of your eye sockets 6–9 times.

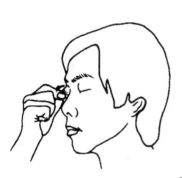

Eyes

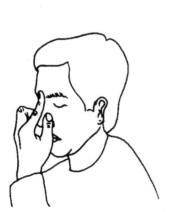
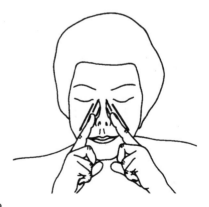

Nose

5. Hold one finger 8 inches from your face. Focus on it without blinking until your eyes tear.

6. Repeat step 1, and rotate your eyeballs behind your palms: 6–9 times clockwise, then counterclockwise.

7. Cup your palms over your closed eyes and inhale. Contract the middle of the anus and pull your eyeballs back into their sockets as you circle your eyeballs: look straight ahead, then to the left, then up, then to the right, and then down.

8. Inhale and contract the left side of the anus and the left sides of the eyeballs, then circle the eyeballs as above.

9. Inhale and contract the front of the anus and the tops of the eyeballs, then circle the eyeballs.

10. Inhale and contract the right side of the anus and the right sides of the eyeballs, then circle them.

Nose

(Pages 40–43)

1. Rub hands briskly together and contract your anus. Stick your thumb and forefinger into your nostrils and move them to the left and right, then up and down 10–20 times.

2. Pinch and rub the bridge of your nose 9–36 times as you inhale and exhale slowly.

3. Massage the mid-nose with the thumb and third finger while your forefinger rests on the bridge. Use index fingers to massage the sides and bottom of the nose.

Sacrum

(Page 67)

1. Bring energy to your hands and contract the back of the anus toward the sacrum.

2. Make fists and use your knuckles to hit both sides of the sacrum alternately. Hit the area of the eight sacral holes first, then the depression at the bottom of the sacrum.

🌀 Ears, Mouth, Face

(Pages 44–54)

1. **Ears:** Place your index fingers behind the ears and your other fingers in front of the ears. Rub the front and back of your ears.

2. With all of your fingers, rub the ear shells, then tug gently on the lobes.

3. Inhale and exhale completely. Put your index fingers in your ears to create a vacuum. Move index fingers back and forth 6–9 times, flexing the eardrums, then pull fingers out with a quick movement.

4. Inhale deeply, then close mouth and pinch nostrils closed. Slowly try to "blow" air out through closed nostrils, then swallow air, causing eardrums to pop. Repeat 2–3 times.

5. Cover ears with palms, pointing your fingers toward the back of your head. Flick your index fingers against the middle fingers, so that the index finger drums on the occipital bone of the skull. Repeat 9 or more times.

6. **Mouth:** Open your mouth and stretch lips tautly. Using the tips of your index, middle, and ring fingers, tap the skin around the upper and lower gums until it feels warm.

7. Massage your upper and lower gums with your tongue.

8. Inhale, then exhale as you press your tongue out and down as far as you can. Then curl the tongue up and in. Press tongue as hard as you can against your palate while contracting the esophagus and the middle of the anus.

9. Relax your lips and click your teeth together lightly. Then clench them hard as you inhale and pull up the middle of the anus. Do this 6–9 times.

10. **Neck:** Separate your thumbs from the fingers and place your hand against your neck. Rapidly wipe the neck from the chin to the base, and repeat with alternating hands 9–36 times.

11. **Shoulders:** Inhale and pull shoulders up toward your ears, while tightening the muscles of the neck and shoulders. Hold a moment, then exhale deeply, letting the shoulders drop down. Repeat 3–9 times.

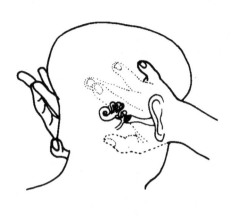

Tapping the eardrums

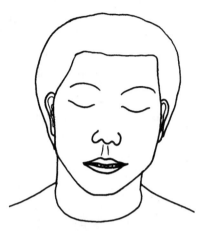

Clicking the teeth

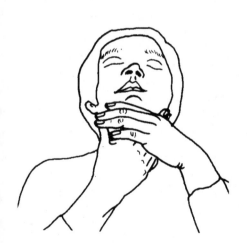

Wiping the neck

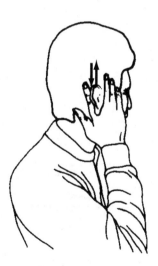

Massaging the scalp

⊙ Hands, Feet, Organs, and Glands
(Pages 21–24, 60–66, 75–79)

1. **Hands:** Bring energy to the hands, and pull the middle of the anus up and toward the front. Massage the palms and the backs of the hands with your thumbs, pressing on bones and major acupuncture points. Massage the fingers, tugging gently on each one.

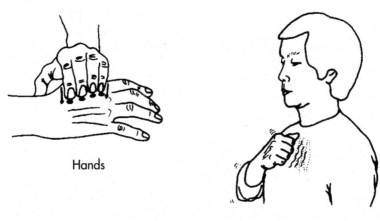

Hands

Thymus

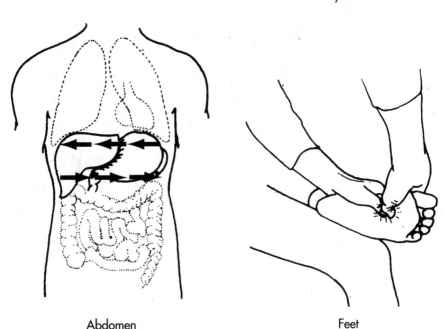

Abdomen

Feet

2. **Thymus and heart:** Bring energy into the hands while contracting the front of the anus and bringing chi toward the thymus. Make a fist, inhale, and thump on the chest (center area, from collarbone to nipples) 6–9 times. Then open your palm and lightly slap the heart area 6–9 times. Do not speak during these exercises.

3. **Lungs and liver:** Contract the anus and lightly slap up and down the right and left lungs. Then contract the right side of anus and slap over the liver, below the rib cage on the right side.

4. **Stomach, spleen, and pancreas:** Slap over the spleen, pancreas, and stomach, then place one palm over the other and rub across the abdomen from right to left (just below ribcage), then left to right (below first line).

5. **Intestines:** With palms together, rub a small circle around the navel (small intestine), first clockwise and then counterclockwise. Then rub a large circle around the whole abdomen (large intestine). Begin on the lower right side and rub up and around in a clockwise direction.

6. **Kidneys:** Make two fists and hit the kidneys (on the back, just above the lowest rib) with the area between the wrist and the knuckles. Rub your palms together briskly until they are warm, then rub them up and down over the kidneys.

7. **Knees:** Prop your leg up on a chair or low table, keeping the knee straight. Bend forward and slap smartly behind the knee 9–18 times, then slap the other leg. Next, massage each kneecap until it is warm. Move the kneecaps with your fingertips: up and down, to the left and right, and then in clockwise and counterclockwise circles.

8. **Feet:** Massage the tops and bottoms of your feet, focusing on painful points until the pain goes away. Be sure to massage Kidney 1/Bubbling Spring. Spread out and separate each toe, then release it. Repeat this 6–9 times, then rub your feet together.

THE SIX HEALING SOUNDS

Lung Exercise: The First Healing Sound
(Pages 21–27)

The lungs are associated with: the large intestine, the metal element, autumn, dryness, white color, pungent flavor, the nose, sense of smell, and the skin, as well as sadness, grief, courage, and justice.

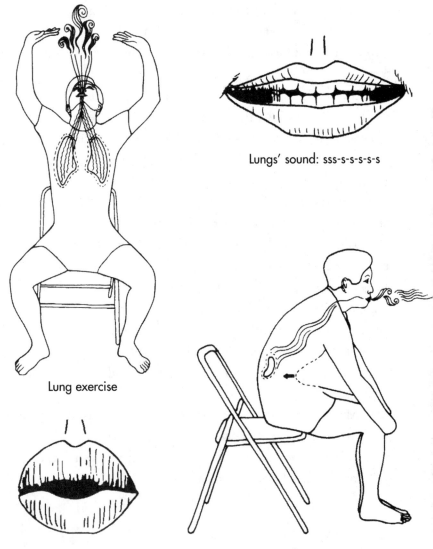

Lung exercise

Lungs' sound: sss-s-s-s-s-s

Kidneys' sound: choo-oo-oo-oo

Kidney exercise

1. While sitting in a chair with your eyes open, rest your hands—palms up—on your thighs.
2. Breathe in slowly and deeply and bring awareness to your lungs. Inhale and raise your arms until hands are at eye level, then rotate palms inward and continue to raise them above your head. Feel all along the arms into your shoulders, and feel the lungs and chest open.
3. Close teeth and make the lungs' sound, sss-s-s-s-s-s, slowly and evenly as you exhale. Picture the lungs exhaling a dark murky color, excess heat, and sick energy, sadness, sorrow, and grief.
4. Float palms down to lungs and then to your lap, facing up. Breathe in pure white light and the quality of righteousness. Close your eyes and smile to your lungs, imagining that you are still making the lungs' sound. Repeat these steps 3–6 times.

⚙ Kidney Exercise: The Second Healing Sound
(Pages 28–33)

The kidneys are associated with: the urinary bladder, the water element, winter, cold, blue color, salty flavor, ears, hearing, and the bones, as well as fear and gentleness.

1. Breathe in slowly and deeply and bring awareness to your kidneys. Bend forward and clasp your hands together around your knees. Pull back on your arms, feeling a stretch on your back, over the kidneys. Look up.
2. Round your lips and make the kidneys' sound, choo-oo-oo-oo, while pulling your mid-abdomen in toward your spine. Blow out a dark, murky color along with any excess heat, wet, sick energy, and fear.
3. Breathe in bright blue energy and the quality of gentleness. Separate your legs and rest your hands, palms up, on your thighs. Close your eyes and smile to your kidneys, imagining that you are still making the kidneys' sound. Repeat these steps 3–6 times.

☯ Liver Exercise: The Third Healing Sound

(Pages 34–40)

The liver is associated with the gallbladder, the wood element, spring, moistness, the color green, the sour flavor, the eyes, and eyesight, as well as with anger, aggression, kindness, and forgiveness.

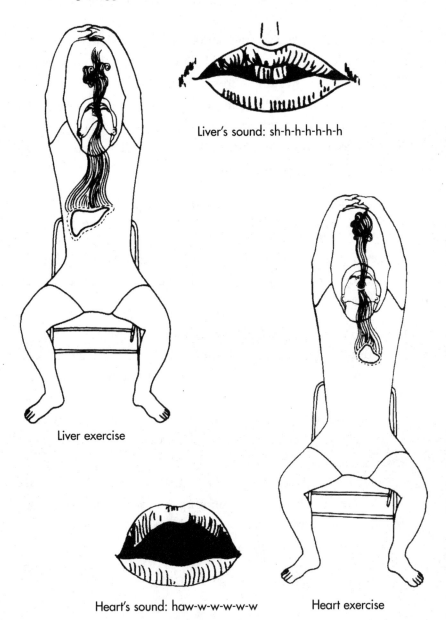

Liver's sound: sh-h-h-h-h-h

Liver exercise

Heart's sound: haw-w-w-w-w

Heart exercise

1. Breathe in slowly and deeply, becoming aware of the liver and its connection to the eyes. Beginning with your arms at your sides, palms out, slowly swing your arms up and over your head, following them with your eyes. Then interlace your fingers and push palms up toward the ceiling, feeling the stretch through arms and shoulders. Bend slightly to the left.

2. Open your eyes wide and exhale the sound sh-h-h-h-h-h-h subvocally, while breathing out a dark murky color filled with excess heat and anger.

3. Press the heels of your palms outward as you lower your shoulders, then place your hands in your lap, palms up. Breathe in a bright green energy and its quality of kindness. Let this energy fill your liver. Close your eyes and smile down to your liver. Repeat these steps 3–6 times.

Heart Exercise: The Fourth Healing Sound
(Pages 41–47)

The heart is associated with the small intestine, the fire element, summer, warmth, the color red, the bitter flavor, the tongue, and speech, as well as with joy, honor, love, creativity, and enthusiasm.

1. Breathe in slowly and deeply while focusing your awareness on your heart. Beginning with palms in your lap, inhale and swing your arms overhead, then clasp fingers together and push palms toward the ceiling, as in the liver exercise. This time, bend slightly to the right.

2. Open your mouth, round your lips, and exhale the sound haw-w-w-w-w-w subvocally, while expelling dark murky energy along with any excess heat, impatience, arrogance, or cruelty.

3. Press palms outward and return hands to your lap, with palms facing upward. Breathe in bright red energy along with its qualities of joy, love, and respect. Smile down to your heart. Repeat these steps 3–6 times.

◉ Spleen Exercise: The Fifth Healing Sound
(Pages 48–53)

The spleen is associated with the stomach and the pancreas, the earth element, Indian summer, dampness, the sweet flavor, the yellow color, the mouth, and taste, as well as with worry, compassion, balance, and openness.

1. Breathe in slowly and deeply, focusing your awareness on the spleen. Inhale and place the fingers of both hands beneath the left side of the ribcage, just below the sternum. Press your fingers inward as you push your middle back outward.
2. Exhale as you round your lips and make the sound of the spleen, who-o-o-o-o-o, from your vocal cords. Expel any excess heat, dampness, worry, or pity.
3. Breathe a bright yellow light into your spleen, stomach, and pancreas, filling them with fairness, compassion, and centeredness. Lower your hands slowly to your lap, palms up, and smile down to your spleen. Repeat these steps 3–6 times.

◉ Triple Warmer Exercise: The Sixth Healing Sound
(Pages 54–58)

The triple warmer consists of the upper warmer (hot: includes the brain, neck, thymus, heart, lungs), the middle warmer (warm: includes the liver, stomach, and spleen), and the lower warmer (cool: includes the intestines, kidneys, and genitals).

1. Lie on your back, close your eyes, and take a deep breath. Inhale fully into all three warmers.
2. Exhale with the sound hee-e-e-e-e-e made subvocally. Imagine a large roller pressing out your breath from the top of your chest and rolling down toward your lower abdomen. Imagine your chest and abdomen are flat, feeling light, bright, and empty.
3. Rest by breathing normally, then repeat these steps 3–6 times.

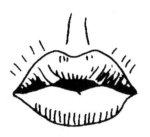

Spleen's sound: who-o-o-o-o-o

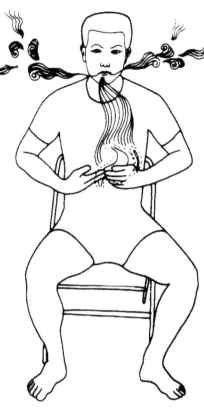

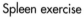

Spleen exercise

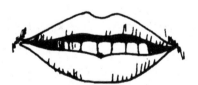

Triple warmer's sound:
hee-e-e-e-e-e

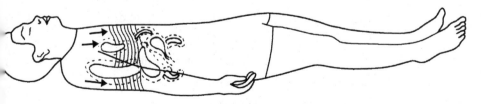

Triple warmer exercise

IRON SHIRT CHI KUNG

⟳ Embracing the Tree

(Pages 72–102)

1. Stand in Embracing the Tree posture (see pages 72–92 of *Iron Shirt Chi Kung*): feet shoulder-width apart and the nine points of the feet in contact with the earth. Tilt your sacrum to open the kua, round the scapulae, sink the chest, tuck the chin in. Extend your arms as if circling around a tree. Keep your thumbs up and your pinkies down, and the rest of the fingers together. Breathe through the mid-eyebrow point, focusing your eyes on your palms. Feel energy 1.5 inches below the navel.

✿ Lower Abdominal Breathing

2. Inhale into area below the navel. Feel air rush into your lungs as the diaphragm drops. Feel the lower abdomen and perineum bulge on all sides.

3. Exhale forcibly through the nose, feeling a ball rolling up your chest. Sink your sternum and press it into the thymus; at the same time, pull up on your anus and genitals. Flatten abdomen toward spine. Repeat lower abdominal breathing 9–18 times.

✿ Iron Shirt Packing Process, first stage

During chi packing, your inhalations should be small sips of air; you will inhale many times before you exhale.

4. Contract your perineum and inhale a bit, pulling the genitals up. Inhale again and pull up the left side of the anus. Pack the left kidney and adrenal gland with chi. Inhale a bit more and tighten the right side of the anus, then pack the right kidney and adrenal gland with chi.

5. Spiral energy at the navel. Circle the energy outward from the navel clockwise 9 times, then counterclockwise 9 times back to the navel center. Spiral your eyes at the same time.

6. With your upper abdomen flat against the spine, inhale into your

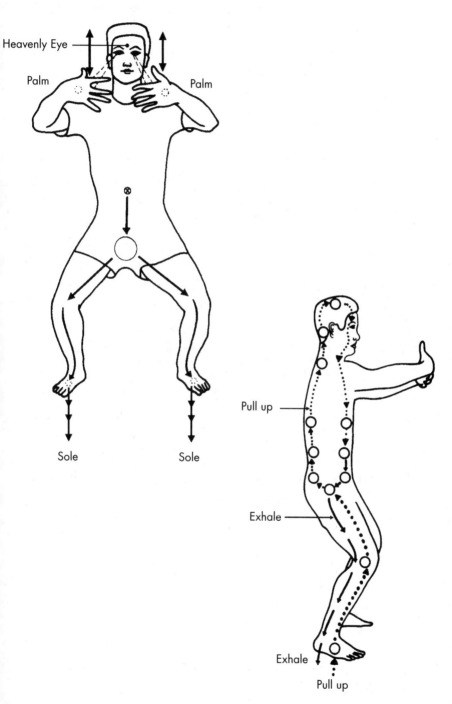

Iron Shirt first posture: Embracing the Tree

lower abdomen. Pull up sex organs and the pelvic and urogenital diaphragms, condensing energy into a chi ball in your lower abdomen.

7. Inhale a bit more, pulling the perineum upward as you pack chi into a ball in the perineal area. Hold the breath for as long as is comfortable.

8. Exhale and relax your whole body. Send energy down through legs into the earth.

🌸 Iron Shirt Packing Process, second stage

9. Press toes and soles of the feet to the floor. Inhale a small breath, pulling earth energy in through the soles. Pull this energy up to the sexual organs, the urogenital and pelvic diaphragms, the left and right sides of the anus, the kidneys, and then into the lower diaphragm. Spiral your eyes and the energy at KD 1 (on the soles of the feet): spiral 9 times clockwise, from KD 1 outward to a diameter of 3 inches, then spiral 9 times counterclockwise back to KD 1.

10. Inhale bringing energy from the toes to the knees. Lock the kneecaps and tighten your legs by rotating the knees outward, feel legs like screws rotating into the ground. Energy collects in the knees.

11. Inhale and pull the genitals and anus up, drawing chi from the knees to the buttocks and then to the perineum. Inhale and pack more chi into the perineum. Feel energy moving down into the perineum from the navel, and up into the perineum from the earth through the legs.

12. Exhale and harmonize your breath with abdominal breathing. Relax and smile down to your organs, then practice Bone Breathing.

🌸 Iron Shirt Packing Process, third stage

13. Pack chi into the kidneys, then gather a chi ball at the navel and bring it into the perineum. Push the chi ball into the ground, then bring it up through the soles to the perineum, joining with the energy from the navel that is already there. Harmonize your breathing.

14. Exhale and flatten the abdomen. Inhale a small bit of air while pulling up the back part of the anus to direct the chi into the sacrum. Activate the sacral pump by tucking the sacrum under slightly, without moving your hips.

15. Bring more kidney energy up from KD 1 to the coccyx and sacrum. Inhale, pulling up the anus and packing chi into the kidneys. Now spiral energy at the sacrum: spiral outward 9 times clockwise, to a diameter of 3 inches. Then circle 9 times counterclockwise back to the center of the sacrum. Feel chi collect in the sacrum.

16. Inhale up to T11. Press T11 and the adrenal glands backward, straightening the curve of the lower back to further activate the sacral pump. Spiral the energy at T11: circle outward 9 times clockwise to a diameter of 3 inches, then circle 9 times counterclockwise back to the center of T11. Feel sacrum and T11 fuse into one channel.

17. Inhale and pull the chi up from T11 to C7. Push from the sternum to tilt C7 back. Tuck your chin, clench teeth, squeeze the temple bones, and press your tongue to the roof of your mouth. When you feel forces pushing at C7, activate the cranial pump. Circle energy at C7: 9 times clockwise out to a diameter of 3 inches, then 9 times inward counterclockwise.

18. Exhale a bit as needed, then inhale and bring the chi up to C1 (Jade Pillow). Spiral energy at C1, outward 9 times clockwise and inward 9 times counterclockwise, until the chi has developed there.

19. Inhale to crown (Crystal Room), the seat of the pineal gland. Look up between eyebrows to help pull chi to the crown. Circle the chi outward 9 times clockwise, then inward 9 times counterclockwise.

20. Pull up and exhale. Do abdominal breathing to harmonize. Place the tongue on the roof of the mouth. Bring energy down from the crown to the third eye, then down to the palate, throat, heart center, and solar plexus. Spiral energy at the solar plexus: outward 9 times clockwise, then inward 9 times counterclockwise. Then bring energy to the navel.

21. Circulate chi in the Microcosmic Orbit for 10–15 minutes. Stand up straight and place your palms over your navel. Practice Bone Breathing and the Power Exercise, then walk around and brush energy downward.

IRON SHIRT CHI KUNG

🌀 Holding the Golden Urn

(Pages 151–61)

Like the previous exercise, this posture uses one breath but many inhalations: you continue inhaling in small sips until you cannot inhale any more, then you exhale.

🌸 Yang Position

1. Assume Embracing the Tree stance with your feet shoulder-width apart. Toes point inward, knees are separated and locked. Forearms are 30 degrees from your sides, shoulders rounded forward, chest sinks down.
2. With palms facing down, lift your forearms and spread your fingers. Pull pinkie fingers outward as far from the other fingers as you can, letting their tendons connect to the tendons of the little toes.
3. Do 9 or 18 rounds of abdominal breathing, then exhale and flatten your abdomen. Inhale and pull up the left and right sides of the anus. Pack chi into and around the kidneys.

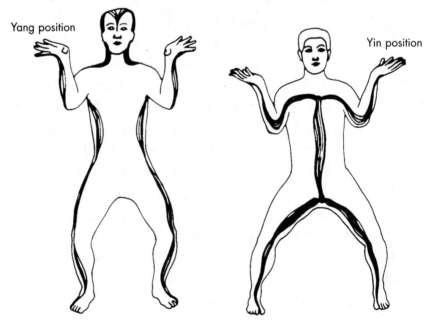

Yang position

Yin position

Iron Shirt second posture: Holding the Golden Urn

4. Inhale and pack chi into the lower abdomen. Contract your anus and pull up on the urogenital diaphragm. Draw energy up from soles of the feet to the sacrum.

5. Inhale and pack chi at the sacrum, tilting it back. Then inhale and pack chi up to T11, pushing T11 back until you feel your spine arched like a flexed bow. Inflate the back with chi pressure, feeling energy rise from Bubbling Spring points to T11. Feel a chi belt stretching from T11 to L2/L3 (Door of Life) and from there to the navel and lower abdomen.

6. Inhale, contracting the anus even more and lifting the genitals. Draw more energy up from feet and pack it into the kidneys and liver.

7. Tilt C7 back, feeling C7, T11, and the sacrum connected as chi inflates the neck. Hold, then inhale and pull up some more, tightening the neck and squeezing the cranial bones. Clench teeth and press tongue to the roof of the mouth.

8. Inhale again, pulling energy up to the base of the skull. Squeeze cranial bones a bit more and push the neck back. Feel the neck and the base of the skull connected to C7, T11, the sacrum, the knees, and the feet. Together these become one flexed bow of strength.

9. Inhale more and tighten, bringing energy up to the crown. Then exhale and relax.

Yin Position

10. Exhale and turn the hands over so that palms are facing up. Rotate wrists outward so the thumbs pull back toward the ears. Wrists should be as close to a 90-degree angle as possible. Stretch the tendons at the wrists by locking the elbows and wrists when you turn your hands. Sink the elbows and round the scapulae.

11. Breathe normally, feeling energy flowing down from the tongue to the solar plexus and navel along the Microcosmic Orbit. Then practice yin breathing by inhaling and exhaling 9 times, exhaling more then you inhale. This will bring energy down the front of the body.

12. Place your hands over the navel and collect chi, then practice Bone Breathing. Walk around, shaking out the legs and brushing down the chest.

Golden Turtle Immersing in Water (Yang)/Water Buffalo Emerging from Water (Yin)

(Pages 161–73)

Yang Position: Golden Turtle Immersing in Water

1. Stand with feet shoulder-width apart and tongue on the roof of the mouth. Do 9 or 18 rounds of abdominal breathing, inhaling more air than you exhale. On the last inhalation, flatten abdomen toward the spine.

2. Inhale as you tighten your fists, fold your forearms against your upper arms, round the back, and sink the chest. Then exhale and bend forward as you straighten your back, so that your whole spine is parallel to the floor. Keeping the forearms folded on the upper arms, expand the scapulae and feel the back energized with chi.

3. Lock the sacrum and open the knees, letting your body weight sink down to the hips, then knees, then feet, then into the ground.

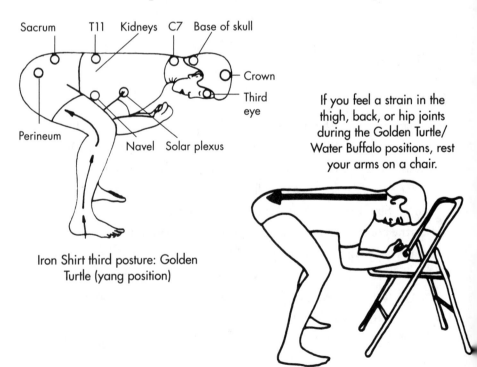

Iron Shirt third posture: Golden Turtle (yang position)

If you feel a strain in the thigh, back, or hip joints during the Golden Turtle/Water Buffalo positions, rest your arms on a chair.

4. Pull energy into the groin area. Tuck in the chin and lock your neck. Press your elbows outward against the insides of the knees while simultaneously pressing the knees inward.

5. Inhale a small sip of air and pack energy into the navel, then inhale a bit more and pack to the lower abdomen.

6. Inhale and pack to the perineum, then pull on the sexual organs more tightly, pulling earth energy up to the perineum. Inhale a bit more and pack to the sacrum, then tilt the sacrum to activate the sacral pump.

7. Inhale and pack to T11, the area of the kidneys and adrenal glands. Press T11 toward the back, then inflate the lower back with chi pressure, energizing the kidneys.

8. Inhale and pack at C7. Tighten the neck and cranial bones, and clench your teeth. Then inhale and pack to the base of the skull, the Jade Pillow. Finally, inhale up to the crown.

9. Now harmonize the breath with abdominal breathing, letting the body relax and flow with chi.

❀ Yin Position: Water Buffalo Emerging from the Water

10. When you have packed energy to the crown in the Golden Turtle exercise, exhale and look upward, releasing the lock in the neck. Extend your arms down in front of you, either your fingertips touching the ground and the backs of your hands facing forward, or your fingertips touching your anus or perineum. Keep the groin open.

11. Rest your tongue on your palate and relax. Inhale more air than you exhale, breathing directly into the groin area. Breathe easily and feel the energy descend to the navel and perineum, activating the lower abdomen and the urogenital and pelvic diaphragms.

12. When your breath has harmonized, close your eyes. Slowly stand up by extending your knees.

13. Work up some saliva, then swallow it down to the navel with a guttural sound. Place your hands over the navel and collect the chi there.

14. Practice Bone Breathing, along with Microcosmic Orbit (optionally). Then walk around, shaking out the legs and brushing down the chest.

⟳ Golden Phoenix Washes Its Feathers

(Pages 173–80)

1. Begin with Iron Shirt Horse stance, arms at your sides. Practice abdominal breathing 9–18 times.

2. Place arms in front of body, palms facing out. Sweep arms out to sides, pulling up through the perineum and anus. Now curl arms under and face your palms toward your armpits, as if gathering something. Point pinkie fingers toward the ceiling. Relax the neck and trapezius muscles, and round your scapulae.

3. Inhale while you pull up the left and right sides of the anus, bringing sexual energy from testicles/ovaries into the kidneys. Pack this energy into kidneys and adrenal glands. Bring palms close to armpits, feeling tendons pull along the insides of the arms to elbows, pinkie fingers, and thumbs.

4. Inhale toward armpits, pulling sexual energy from testicles/ovaries to the kidneys and up to the spleen (left side) and the liver (right side). Pack chi into these organs, then wrap chi around them. Inhale and bring hands as close to the armpits as possible, while pulling sexual energy up to the heart and lungs.

5. While keeping the anus contracted and genitals pulled up, exhale. Turn palms to face outward. Push from the sternum to C7 while extending your arms and making the lungs' sound (sss-s-s-s-s-s) releasing organ pressure.

6. With arms fully extended, inhale as you contract the middle of the anus and pull sexual organs up. Form beaks by gathering fingers to the thumbs in a small point. Inhale again as you pull the beaks inward from the elbows and contract the middle part of the anus. Inhale again, pulling the beaks closer to your body, further tightening the anus and genitals. Pull elbows and wrists to chest, beaks pointed out.

7. Exhale, making the kidneys' sound (choo-oo-oo-oo). At the same time, open the beaks and extend your arms straight down in front of you, spreading the fingers wide. When arms reach hips, lock your elbows and rotate the hands outward, keeping the fingers spread.

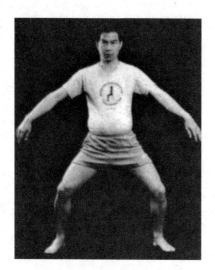

Sweep arms to sides.

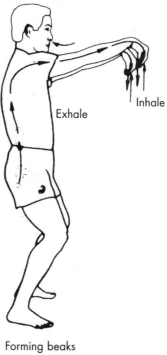

Inhale

Exhale

Forming beaks

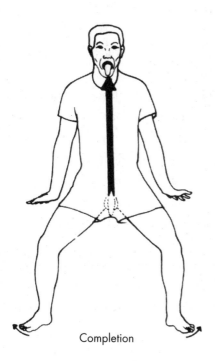

Completion

Golden Phoenix Washes Its Feathers

8. Exhale again while extending the finger tendons (especially pinkies and thumbs) and spreading the toes. At the same time, extend your tongue out toward the chin as far as you can and look at your nose. Finally, bring your feet together in small "steps" by turning your big toes inward, then your heels.

9. Repeat this exercise 2 more times: the first time replace the lungs' sound in step 5 with the liver's sound (sh-h-h-h-h-h) and the kidneys' sound in step 7 with the heart's sound (haw-w-w-w-w-w." The second time use the spleen's sound in step 5 (who-o-o-o-o-o) and the triple warmer's sound in step 7 (hee-e-e-e-e-e).

10. Spread the fingers and extend the arms. Relax and feel chi spread out to all the tendons of the hands, arms, legs, and tongue. Collect energy at the navel, then do Bone Breathing.

Iron Bridge

(Pages 183–90)

1. Stand with knees straight and feet 12 inches apart, toes pointed straight ahead. With your hands slightly in front of the body, form a circle with the thumb and index finger of each hand.

2. Yang position: Begin abdominal breathing, then exhale and flatten the abdomen. Inhale to full capacity, then move your hands up along your back, with palms facing upward and fingers reaching toward the scapulae. Open your chest and abdomen, and tighten your thighs and buttocks.

3. Clench your teeth and arch backward, beginning with the head, which should be supported by the neck muscles. Look backward, stretching the fasciae at the front of the neck, which will then lift the chest and abdomen.

4. Push the pelvis forward, keeping the thighs and pelvis tight. Do not overstretch. Squeeze thumb and index fingers together, tightening the muscles in the arms and shoulders. Hold your breath and maintain this position for 30–60 seconds.

5. Yin position: Exhale as you straighten up and bring arms to the front. Slowly bend forward from the hips until your head is down and your hands are dangling. Knees can be lightly bent.

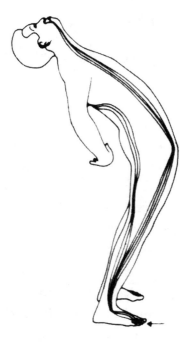

Iron Bridge yang position

6. Come up slowly and stand still, collecting the energy. Practice Bone Breathing.

Iron Bar

(Pages 191–94)

1. Place two chairs across from each other. Put your feet and lower legs on one chair, with toes pointed down and away from you. Lay your head and shoulders on the other chair. (If this exercise is difficult, bring your arms overhead, and rest them on the chair beneath your head.)
2. Maintain a straight back, and avoid stressing the lower spine by tightening the buttocks and feeling the sacrum squeeze down. Breathe normally from the abdomen.
3. Slowly lower your buttocks and feet to the floor and sit with your tongue on the roof of your mouth. Let the energy flow in the Microcosmic Orbit.

HEALING LOVE THROUGH THE TAO
Cultivating Female Sexual Energy

❂ Ovarian Breathing
(Pages 60–83)

Ovarian Breathing can be practiced sitting, standing, or lying down.

Sitting: Sit on a chair so that your weight is distributed to your legs and buttocks. Cover your vagina and perineum with comfortable underwear or loose clothing. If needed, press a small ball against your clitoris. Your feet should be flat on the floor and your palms on your knees.

Standing: Stand up straight and relaxed with feet shoulder-width apart and your hands at your sides.

Lying on right side: Use a pillow to raise your head 3–4 inches. Place your right thumb behind your ear and fold it slightly forward; keep the other fingers in front of the ear. Rest your left hand on the outer left thigh. Bend the left knee slightly and rest it on top of the right leg, which should be straight.

1. Round your neck and shoulders slightly, and place your tongue on the roof of your mouth. Inhalations during this practice should be small sips of air; there may be many inhalations for each exhalation.
2. Collect ovary energy in the Ovarian Palace by rubbing your ovaries in spirals. At the same time, "breathe" with your PC muscle, using it to gently close and open the vagina. When you feel energy manifesting— as warmth, tightness, tingling, etc.—inhale and bring that energy to the Ovarian Palace.
3. Inhale and contract the vagina, pulling it downward as you pull up on the front part of the perineum. This will bring the energy down from the Ovarian Palace to the perineum. Then inhale short sips and close the vagina tightly, collecting energy at the front part of the perineum. Exhale.
4. Inhale and exhale 9 times, drawing energy from the Ovarian Palace to the front part of the perineum.

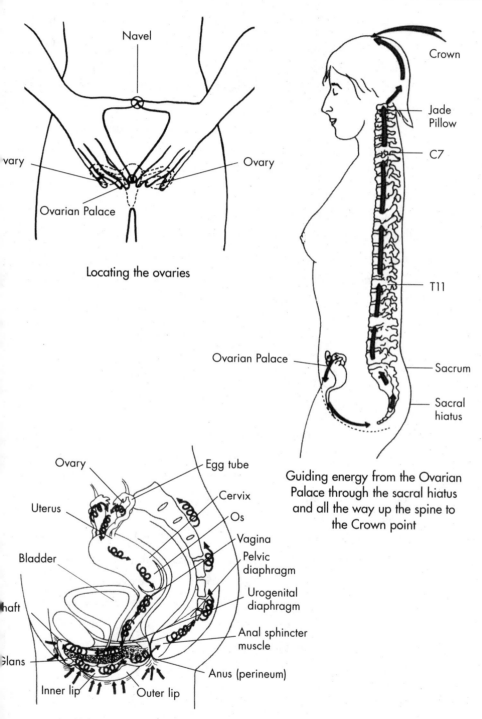

Navel

Ovary

Ovary

Ovarian Palace

Locating the ovaries

Crown

Jade Pillow

C7

T11

Ovarian Palace

Sacrum

Sacral hiatus

Guiding energy from the Ovarian Palace through the sacral hiatus and all the way up the spine to the Crown point

Ovary

Egg tube

Uterus

Cervix

Os

Bladder

Vagina

Pelvic diaphragm

Urogenital diaphragm

Shaft

Anal sphincter muscle

Glans

Anus (perineum)

Inner lip

Outer lip

Energy flow during Ovarian Breathing

5. Repeat steps 3 and 4, then bring the energy through the sacral hiatus and into the sacrum; hold it there. Activate the sacral pump. Repeat 9 times.

6. Repeat steps 3 and 4 a total of 4 more times, bringing the energy to T11, then C7, the Jade Pillow, and the crown. After each repetition, return your energy to the ovaries, while leaving a part of your attention on the energy collected at the perineum.

7. When you have filled the Crown point with creative sexual energy, let it fill your brain. Then spiral the energy in your brain outward in counterclockwise circles 36 times. Then spiral inward 36 times clockwise.

8. Keeping your tongue on your palate, let the warm energy flow down to the mid-eyebrow point and throat to the heart center. Let the heart fill with energy, then draw it down through the solar plexus to the navel. Collect energy at the navel by spiraling outward 36 times counterclockwise, then spiraling inward clockwise 24 times.

⟳ Ovarian Compression
(Pages 89–95)

1. In a sitting or standing position, inhale slowly through your nose, compressing the air in your throat until you can inhale no further.

2. Swallow strongly to the solar plexus, collecting the energy there like a ball. Press this chi ball down to the navel, then down to the pelvic region.

3. Contract the abdominal muscles downward and pack and compress the ovaries. Squeeze the lips of the vagina so that it feels like it is blowing up like a balloon. As energy is driven into the ovaries, you will feel a flush of heat. Forcibly compress the energy into the ovaries for as long as you can, feeling the heat flow up the spine to your head.

4. Exhale and relax completely, then take quick short breaths through your nostrils. Rotate your waist several times.

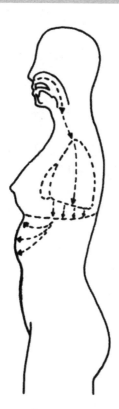

Swallow air down to
the solar plexus.

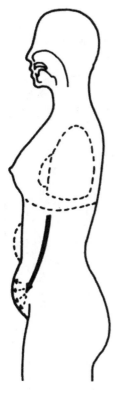

Push air down to the
lower abdomen.

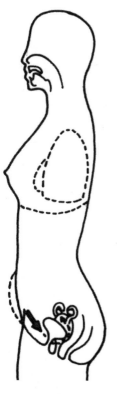

Press air down to
the vagina.

✪ The Orgasmic Upward Draw
(Pages 96–145)

1. Sit with your feet flat on the floor. Stimulate your breasts and direct the sexual energy down to your ovaries. Expand it in the ovaries and genitals, then concentrate it in the Ovarian Palace.

2. When you are near or in the midst of an orgasm, inhale deeply through the nose. At the same time, clench your jaw and both fists, claw your feet, tighten the cranial pump at the back of your neck, and press your tongue firmly to the roof of your mouth.

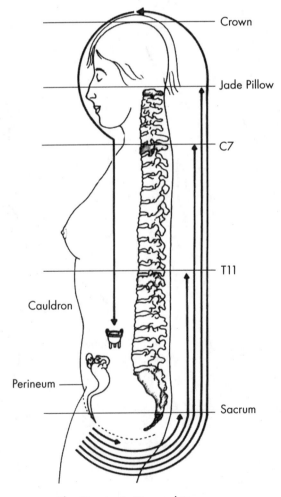

The Orgasmic Upward Draw

3. Inhale again, drawing up the entire anus and genital region—especially the front part of the perineum. Pull the energy from the Ovarian Palace to the perineum by clenching your vaginal lips together to squeeze the clitoris. Hold breath then inhale again. Hold breath again while you contract and pull down the front part of the anus, pulling energy down from the ovaries to collect at the perineum.

4. Inhale without exhaling, then clench and pull up your sexual region 9 times, holding energy at the front part of the perineum. Exhale and release all the muscles of the body.

5. Repeat steps 1–3 again, this time continuing to pull the energy up through the perineum and into the coccyx and sacrum. Contract the middle and back parts of the anus as you do this. Arch your sacrum back and outward to activate the sacral pump. Hold the energy here and inhale 3–9 times, creating contractions to pull the energy from the Ovarian Palace and sexual organs. Then exhale and relax.

6. Repeat steps 1–3 again, now drawing the sexual energy up through the perineum and sacrum to T11. Hold the energy at T11, then add the energy from the Ovarian Palace by inhaling and contracting 9 times without exhaling, Then exhale and relax, mentally guiding energy from the Ovarian Palace to T11.

7. Repeat steps 1–3 again, drawing the energy all the way up to C7. At C7, push the top of the sternum back toward the spine to increase the pumping of energy and to activate the thymus.

8. Repeat the same steps again, this time drawing energy to the Jade Pillow. To activate the cranial pump there, tuck the chin in. Clench your teeth, squeeze the back of your skull, and press your tongue hard against your palate to increase the pumping action.

9. Repeat again, now drawing energy to the Crown point, Pai Hui. Turn your eyes and all senses to the top of the skull and press your tongue firmly to your palate. Practice 9 hard contractions and continue to inhale, each time pulling energy from the Ovarian Palace to the crown. With your mind, eyes, and senses, spiral the energy at the crown 9–36 times clockwise, then counterclockwise.

10. Rest and allow the energy to enter your brain. Let extra energy run down the Functional Channel to the mid-eyebrow point, nose, throat, heart center, solar plexus, and navel.
11. Massage your breasts and genitals.

Four Stages of the Orgasmic Draw Practice
(Pages 101–2)

1. **Stage one:** Use all the muscles of the fists, jaws, neck, feet, perineum, buttocks and abdomen to help activate the sacral and cranial pumps and push the energy upward.
2. **Stage two:** Use less tension in the fists, jaws, and feet, relying instead on the chi muscle of the perineum to activate the sacral and cranial pumps.
3. **Stage three:** Use less tension in the chi muscle and more mind power to activate the pumps.
4. **Stage four:** No need for muscle contractions; you will use pure mind control to command the ovaries and compel the sexual energy to move upward.

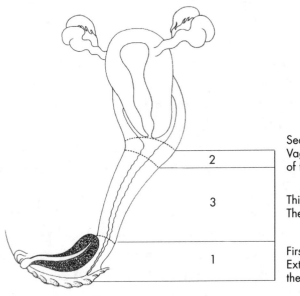

Second section:
Vaginal canal in front of the cervix

Third section:
The middle vaginal canal

First section:
External vaginal orifice to the front of the vaginal canal

The three sections of the vagina

◯ Egg Exercise

(Pages 146–64)

1. Insert the egg into your vagina large end first. Stand in Horse stance and contract the first section of the vaginal canal—the muscles that close the vaginal orifice.

2. Inhale and contract the muscles immediately in front of your cervix while keeping the first set of muscles contracted.

3. Using the muscles in the middle of the vaginal canal, lightly squeeze the egg. Inhale and squeeze harder, then move the egg up and down. When you are out of breath, exhale and rest.

4. Use the top set of muscles—those in front of the cervix—to move the egg left and right, then rest. Now use the bottom set of muscles (controlling the vaginal orifice) to move the egg left and right.

5. Use the top set of muscles, then the bottom set, to tilt the egg up and down. Combine all of the movements, then slide the egg up to touch the cervix and down to the vaginal orifice. Release.

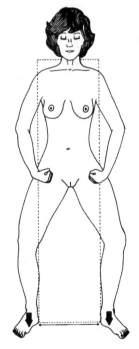

Horse stance for the Egg Exercise

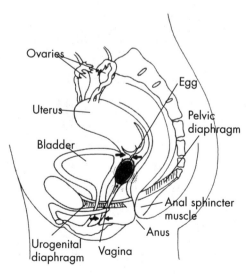

Egg Exercise

HEALING LOVE THROUGH THE TAO

Dual Cultivation

(Pages 203–9)

1. Lie on your side facing your partner. Use foreplay to bring one or both partners to the boiling point. One or both partners place the right palm on your partner's sacrum with your middle finger touching the tip of the coccyx. Place your left hand on the partner's Door of Life.

   Feel sexual energy move upward from the sexual region to the sacrum and kidneys. Inhale to pack and wrap the kidneys with healing, creative energy.

2. When sexual energy is low, practice shallow thrusting: 3, 6, or 9 shallow thrusts to one deep thrust. Build the energy, then embrace quietly for a while.

3. With your right hand still holding the sacrum, move your left hand to T11. Hold this position until both partners feel the energy move up to T11.

4. Continue building sexual energy and moving it up the spine: in succession touch the liver and spleen point (below and between the scapulae), the heart point, C7, Jade Pillow, and the crown. Build the energy before each step, and hold it for a moment afterward.

5. At the Jade Pillow point, feel the sacral and cranial pumps activating. At the Crown point, feel energy fill the brain, then shower down the Functional Channel to the tongue, heart, and navel.

6. Look into your partner's eyes/soul, exchanging healing energy like magnets. Rub noses and tongues, feeling cosmic energy flowing between you.

7. If possible without causing an orgasm, the woman can lightly squeeze and hold her vagina, sending the healing sexual energy wherever her partner needs it.

8. Bring energy to the heart, then collect energy at the navel.

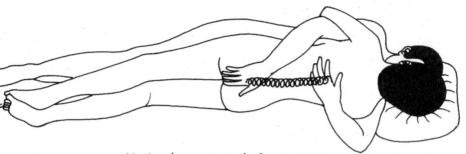

Moving the energy to the heart point

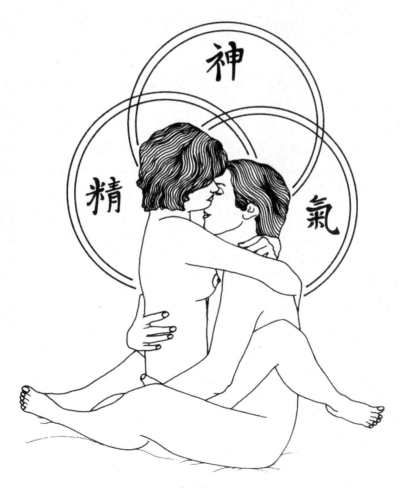

Dual Cultivation

🌀 Valley Orgasm

(Pages 210–41)

1. Make love actively in any position. Use 3, 6, or 9 shallow thrusts for each deep thrust.
2. Stop thrusting on the verge of orgasm. Women do the Orgasmic Upward Draw and men do the Big Draw to bring the energy up to the crown.
3. Embrace and synchronize your breathing, then each partner open the Microcosmic Orbit.
4. Exchange power by circulating your energy back and forth between you gently. Feel the energy build in your lower tan tien, then move it upward in a wave toward your solar plexus and heart tan tien.
5. When your arousal has diminished by about 50 percent, thrust again to build up more energy. Keep the urogenital diaphragm closed and stop before ejaculation.
6. Repeat steps 4 and 5 several times, each time bringing the energy up to increasingly higher centers—the throat center, the third eye center, and the Crown point.
7. Rest and absorb the energy for 10–20 minutes. Then collect energy at your navel.

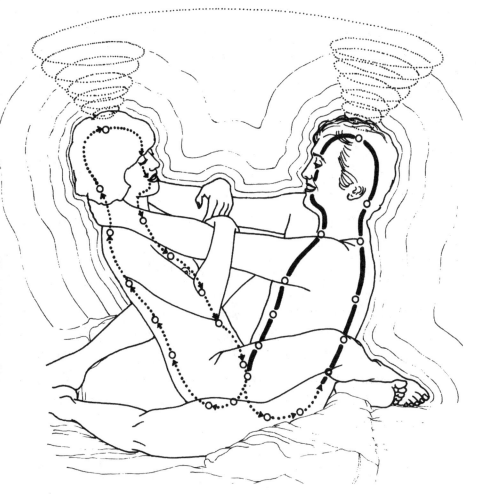

Exchanging yin and yang energies through the Microcosmic Orbit

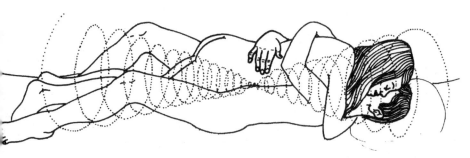

Absorbing yin and yang after lovemaking

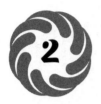

Level Two

Level Two explores the basic practices of the Universal Healing Tao system that appear in the following titles from Destiny Books: *Bone Marrow Nei Kung, Fusion of the Five Elements,* and *The Inner Structure of Tai Chi.*

Collectively, the Level Two practices begin the development of the energy body. Every time you do these practices you are building an energetic tank that will help you travel safely in the realms of the great beyond.

BONE MARROW NEI KUNG

Theory: In order to grow bone and build blood—and thereby increase your longevity—you need to activate the marrow. This means working with your bones, which are the strongest part of your body. Composed in part of crystal, these factories of blood and marrow contain the body's densest forms of chi.

Concept: The Bone Marrow Nei Kung practices stimulate the bone marrow with wire and rattan hitting techniques, bone breathing and compression techniques, and genital massage and weight lifting. Bone Breathing uses the power of the mind, along with deep, relaxed inhalations, to establish an inward flow of external energy through the fingertips and toes. After external energy has been breathed into a particular area, muscle contractions are used to force the combined energies into the bones to burn the fat out of the marrow.

While Bone Breathing is a mental process used in conjunction with long, soft breath cycles, Bone Compression is a physical process of contracting the muscles, thereby squeezing chi into the bones. The purpose of the Sexual Energy Massage is to release Ching Chi—which actually refers to the combination of sexual energy and the sexual hormones—from the genitals so that it can be disseminated throughout the body and absorbed into the bones. Although the combined energies from sexual and external sources are used to burn fat out of the bones, only Ching Chi can regenerate bone marrow.

The hitting techniques can be employed to detoxify the body, stimulate the lymphatic and nervous systems, or compress chi into the bones.

Purpose: Bone Marrow Nei Kung is the third level of the Iron Shirt Chi Kung practices. Its methods of absorbing energy into the bones revives the bone marrow, rejuvenates the organs and glands, and reverses the effects of aging, increasing your health and longevity.

FUSION OF THE FIVE ELEMENTS

Theory: The fusion practices teach us to transform our negative emotions into more positive forms of energy. Typically, when we get angry we unleash our anger on somebody else, but the Taoists say: Why give this precious energy away? Positive and negative energy are still energy, so why not use it? If we transform our negative energies internally, then we can balance and heal our bodies. This kind of transformation is the key to the Fusion formulas.

Concept: The Fusion formulas are like composting machines: with them, we can turn our negative energy into positive life force. We build this composting machine with the four pakuas, then form a pearl with the excess internal energy gleaned from Balancing the Inner Climate and Connecting the Senses. By circulating this pearl we open thirty-two energy channels inside and outside the body. Next, we practice the advanced fusion formulas (Protective Animals, Energy Body, and Planetary Forces) to build an energetic protection field around the body.

Purpose: With daily meditation practice you can establish and maintain an energetic transformation machine and protection field to balance, transform, and heal your body. Once this vortex is in place, it will automatically transform any imbalanced energy that you encounter—internally or externally—so that negative energies will not impede your continued growth.

THE INNER STRUCTURE OF TAI CHI

Theory: These practices explore the first Tai Chi Chi Kung form. Unlike regular Tai Chi, which is just a kind of movement, Tai Chi Chi Kung involves working with internal energies as you move within the form, implementing the beginning Iron Shirt principles.

Concept: This is a Yang style form with thirteen movements in four directions. It begins in the north and moves counterclockwise 360 degrees, then returns clockwise 360 degrees to the original position. With daily practice you will build up a complete energetic defense system, whose postures and strikes become part of your muscle memory.

Purpose: Once you learn the form according to the ten-thousand-practice rule (by doing it ten thousand times), you know it completely; it activates your molecular memory and becomes incorporated into your energy body. When you leave your physical body, you will take the form's postures and strikes with you to the next plane.

BONE MARROW NEI KUNG

⊙ Wire Rod Hitting: Intro, Arms, and Legs

(Pages 110–36)

❈ Preliminary Strokes

Hitting of these four areas should be practiced both before and after the main hitting sequence. Rest and practice Bone Breathing in between rounds.

1. **Tan tien/lower abdomen:** Find the point located 3 inches below the navel and hit 3 times. Then pack energy into this point and hit it 3 more times. Rest and absorb chi.

2. **Ming Men:** Hit the Ming Men point (on the spine, opposite the navel) 3 times. Pack this area—including the two kidneys—by drawing energy up from the perineum while pulling up the left and right sides of the anus. Pack and hit 3 times, then rest and absorb chi.

3. **Inside of the elbow:** Hit the inside of either elbow 3 times, then rest and repeat. Then repeat this procedure on the other arm.

4. **Back of the knee:** Hit the back of one knee 3 times, then rest and breathe energy into the bones. Hit 3 more times and rest again. Repeat this sequence on the other leg.

❈ Lines on the Arms

(Pages 120–24)

5. **Inside elbow, middle finger line:** Raise one arm, keeping the palm up and fingers extended. Hit the inside of the elbow 3 times, then continue hitting as you move the striker down the inside of the forearm to the tip of the middle finger. Then reverse direction, hitting your way up the inner arm, across the inner elbow, to reach the shoulder at the front of the collarbone. Rest and absorb the chi.

6. **Inside elbow, thumb line:** With your arm extended above the shoulder and palm facing up, hit the point on the inside of the elbow that is in line with the thumb. Hit down the inside of the forearm to the

tip of the thumb, then hit back up the arm—through the inner elbow to the clavicle. Rest and absorb chi.

7. **Outside elbow, index finger line:** Raise the arm above the shoulder with your palm facing down and the thumb slightly lower than the pinkie. Hit the point on the outside of the forearm that is at the level of the elbow and on a line with the index finger. Hit the point 3 times, then hit down the outside of the forearm toward the tip of the index finger. Then return along the same line to the shoulder. Rest and absorb chi.

8. **Outside elbow, pinkie finger line:** Lower your arm with the palm facing outward. The thumb should be pointing toward the floor and the pinkie should be the highest point of the hand. Hit the point on the outside of the elbow that is in line with the pinkie finger. Hit 3 times, then hit down the ulna bone and across the wrist to the outside tip of the pinkie finger. Return along the same line to the back of the shoulder, near the outside edge of the scapula. Rest and absorb chi.

9. Repeat steps 5–8 on the other arm.

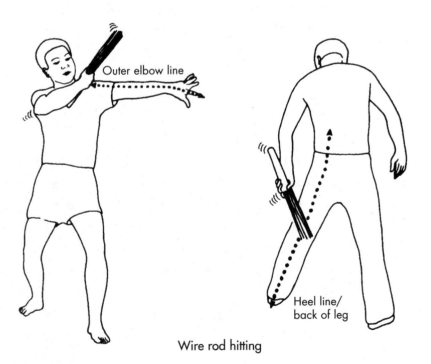

Outer elbow line

Heel line/
back of leg

Wire rod hitting

❁ Lines of the Leg
(Pages 125–28)

10. **Back of the leg, heel line:** Move the right leg forward and bend it slightly, while the left leg remains straight. With hitting device in the left hand, hit the back of your left knee 3 times, then pack and hit from the left buttock down to the heel of the left foot. Return back up the leg to a point on the back 3 inches directly to the left of Ming Men. Rest and absorb chi.

11. **Outside of leg, fourth toe line:** Maintain the stance from step 10 and hit the point on the outside of your leg that is at a level with the bottom of your kneecap. Hit this point 3 times, then pack and hit the outside of the leg from the hip down to the outer edge of the ankle, ending at the tip of the fourth toe. Return up the leg along the same line. Rest and absorb chi.

12. **Inside of the leg, big toe line:** With your feet parallel, move your left leg one half-step to the side. Men should cover their genitals with the right hand. Pack and hit 3 times the point on the inner side of the leg at the level of the bottom of the kneecap. Then, hit from a point near the genitals down the inside of the leg to the tip of the big toe. Avoid hitting the ankle bone directly. Return up this same line to a point near the genitals, then rest and absorb the chi.

13. **Front of leg, middle toe line:** Locate the center of the inguinal groove on the front of the leg where the leg meets the body. Hit down the midline of the leg from this centerpoint, skipping over the knee and ending at the tip of the middle toe. Gently hit the bony top of the foot an additional 3 times. Return back up this line to the inguinal groove, then hit the back of the knee 3 times. Rest and absorb the energy, then repeat steps 11–13 on the right leg.

14. Sit on a chair and hit the Bubbling Spring point on the sole of each foot 9–36 times.

☯ Wire Rod Hitting: Trunk and Head
(Pages 112–19)

❀ Abdominal Lines

1. **Center line:** In Horse stance, inhale a small sip of air while pulling up the genitals and the pelvic and urogenital diaphragms. Direct chi to the navel, then spiral, pack, and squeeze the chi there, striking over the navel 3 times. Continue down this center line to the pubic bone, packing and hitting, then follow the same line back up to the solar plexus. Exhale, relax, and absorb the chi.

2. **Left side of abdomen, interior line:** Locate the interior line on the left side of the abdomen, 1.5 inches to the left of the centerline. Spiral, pack, and hit the chi along this line from the navel to the pubic bone, then up the same line to the diaphragm. Exhale, relax, and absorb the chi.

3. **Left side of abdomen, exterior line:** Locate the exterior left abdomen line 3 inches from the centerline, and spiral, pack, and hit the chi there. With the left hand raised, used the right hand to follow the exterior line down to a point near the hip, then back up to just below the rib cage. Exhale, relax, and absorb the chi.

4. **Right side of abdomen, interior and exterior lines:** Repeat steps 2 and 3 on the right side of the abdomen.

5. **Sides of the trunk:** Raise the left hand overhead and hit the left side of the body with the right hand. Begin at the floating rib—at the level of the navel—and hit down the far left side of the body to the hip, then back up the side to the armpit, then down again to the floating rib. Exhale and absorb the chi, then repeat on the right side using your left hand.

6. **Rib cage:** Inhale and pack chi into the left side while pulling up the left side of the anus. Beginning at the bottom of the sternum, use the hitting device in your right hand to gently hit the lowest left rib from the sternum outward to the left side. Move up about 1.5 inches and hit along the next rib, from the sternum outward. Continue moving

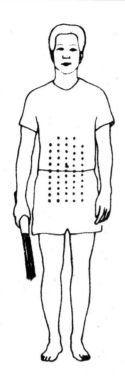

Five lines of the abdomen

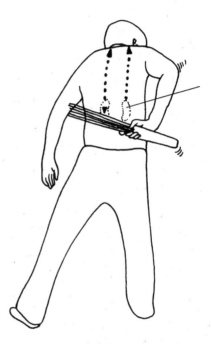

Back lines

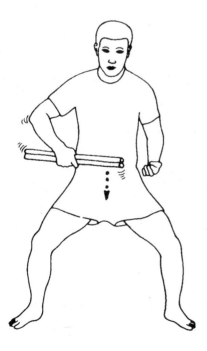

Hitting with rattan sticks

up about 1.5 inches to hit each rib. Then switch sides, and hit the right side of the rib cage with your left hand.

7. **Sternum and collarbones:** Gently hit the sternum from the bottom to the top, then hit along each collarbone to the shoulder. Exhale, relax, and absorb the chi.

✿ Back and Head

It is easier to have a partner hit the lines of the back for you.

8. **Back lines:** Inhale and pack chi into the kidneys and back. First, hit the point 3 inches directly to the left of Ming Men 3 times. Then round the scapulae and sink the chest. Pack and hit the left kidney gently, then hit vertically all the way up to the neck. Pull your chin in, clench your teeth, and press your tongue to your palate as you reach the base of the skull. Return down this line to a point to the left of the sacrum, then go back up to the starting point. Rest and absorb the chi, then repeat on the right side, beginning at a point 3 inches to the right of Ming Men.

9. **Head:** Pull back the chin, clench your teeth, and press your tongue to your palate, then gently tap around the hairline. Never hit the top or the crown of the head. Then lightly tap around the outside edges of the lower jaw.

◉ Rattan Stick Hitting
(Pages 128–36)

Practice after any other hitting methods, and do not use any chi-packing practices during Rattan Stick Hitting. Never hit the sacrum, spinal cord, or joints with rattan sticks.

1. Hit muscle areas, navel, abdominal lines, and sides. Sticks should be applied very lightly to shins and kidneys. Relax and absorb chi.

BONE MARROW NEI KUNG

Bone Breathing

(Pages 28–47)

Beginning students may wish to practice with one limb at a time, while more advanced students can breathe into two limbs, or four at a time.

1. Raise your hands, and gently pull up the genitals and anus with each breath. Bend and sink the elbows, feeling a coolness in the tips of the fingers. This coolness will attract warm external energies. Inhale a long, gentle breath, and pull in the entire hand, feeling the warmth of the energy as it enters your index finger first, then the other fingers and the thumb. Then exhale and slowly extend your hand, feeling the energy leave the extended fingers.

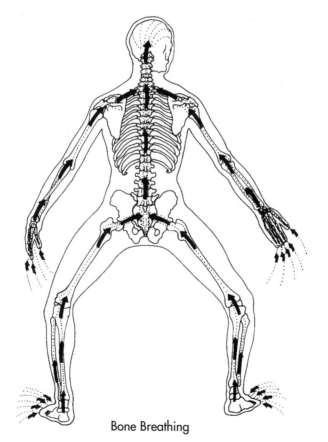

Bone Breathing

2. Inhale through all of your fingertips, filling the knuckles with chi. Lightly pull up genitals as you draw energy in. Inhale and hold for a while, feeling the fingers expand with energy, then exhale.

3. Inhale into the small bones of the wrist, then into the radius and ulna of the forearm. Hold each breath and feel the bones expand, then exhale. Inhale through the fingers, wrists, and forearms to the humerus bones of the upper arms. Exhale and continue breathing in and out of the bones, then breathe normally and rest.

4. Inhale again through the fingers, hands, forearms, and upper arms, keeping your elbows and shoulders dropped. Exhale, then inhale again into the scapulae and C7. Hold the energy there, continuing to breathe in and out of the bones, then rest.

5. Create a sensation of coolness in the toes. Inhale and draw warm external energies into the toes and feet. Exhale and release. Pull up on the genitals slightly as you draw the chi into the tibia and fibula bones of the lower legs. Exhale and release, then inhale again, drawing energy into the femur bones, then the hips, and then the sacrum. Exhale.

6. In Embracing the Tree posture, inhale into both hands and feet simultaneously, drawing energy all the way up the arms to the shoulders and scapulae, and up the legs to the hip bones and sacrum. Then combine the arm and leg energy in the middle of the spine (T11). Inhale and draw this combined energy to the shoulders, then to C7, the base of the skull (Jade Pillow), and into the head. Hold your breath for a moment, then exhale.

7. Inhale energy into the head as in step 6, then bring it from the head back down the spinal cord to C7. From there, spiral energy throughout the head and the facial bones, then spread from the back of the collarbones and the back of the ribs around to the sternum. Then exhale and release.

⚙ Bone Compression

(Pages 47–61)

Bone Compression follows the same sequence as Bone Breathing, but the circulation of energy is different; Bone Compression involves spiraling the incoming chi, then packing it between the muscles before squeezing it into the bones.

1. Inhale into fingers, wrists, and ulna and radius bones, holding the intake from each breath. Spiral energy around these bones— clockwise spiral on the right arm, counterclockwise on the left arm.
2. After spiraling, inhale again, and mentally pack the energy between the muscles and the bones. Pull up lightly on the anus and genitals. Continue packing until the arms feel swollen and heavy with chi.
3. Use hard muscular contractions to squeeze the accumulated energy into the bones. Feel heat in the marrow, and squeeze a little more to reach the deeper parts of the bone. Hold breath for a moment, then exhale.
4. Inhale energy into the arms, shoulders, scapulae, and collarbones.

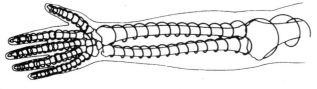

a. Spiraling the energy around the bones

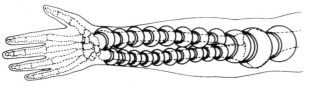

b. Packing energy between the muscles and bones

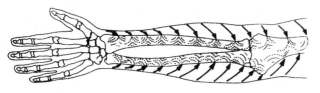

c. Squeezing the energy into the bones

Bone Compression

Then spiral, pack, and squeeze the energy into the bones. Then exhale and release. Inhale again and bring energy through the arms, shoulders, and scapulae into the spine down to T11, where the energy from the upper body combines with that of the lower body. Spiral, pack, and squeeze.

5. Inhale energy into both legs, drawing it through the feet, legs, and hips and into the sacrum. Then spiral, pack, and squeeze this energy into the bones. Inhale again through the feet, legs, and sacrum, bringing energy up the spine to the first lumbar vertebra. Hold the energy and inhale again, packing into the sacrum and spine, then squeezing the muscles of the legs, hips, buttocks, and lower back. Hold the contraction with your breath, then release it as you exhale.

6. Inhale and spiral energy from the legs and arms to meet at T11. From here, spiral the energy further up the spine into the neck and head. With your tongue against your palate, spiral energy throughout the cranium, then pack and clench your teeth to squeeze the energy into the cranial bones.

7. Inhale and spiral chi from the spine through all of the ribs simultaneously. Pack and squeeze into the ribs and sternum by sinking the chest and squeezing the chest muscles. Exhale and relax, feeling heat moving through your bones. Shake out your body so the energy does not get congested.

For advanced practice, you can spiral, pack, and squeeze energy into the whole body in one breath.

BONE MARROW NEI KUNG

⊙ Testicle Breathing

(Pages 204–5)

Testicle Breathing can be practiced sitting, standing, or lying down.

Sitting: Sit on a chair so that your weight is distributed to your legs and buttocks. Cover your genitals with comfortable underwear or loose clothing. Your feet should be flat on the floor, and your palms on your knees.

Standing: Stand up straight and relaxed with feet shoulder-width apart and your hands at your sides.

Lying on right side: Use a pillow to raise your head 3–4 inches. Place your right thumb behind your ear and fold it slightly forward; keep the other fingers in front of the ear. Rest your left hand on the outer left thigh. Bend the left knee slightly and rest it on top of the right leg, which should be straight.

1. Round your neck and shoulders slightly, and place your tongue on the roof of your mouth. Inhalations during this practice should be small sips of air; there may be many inhalations for each exhalation.

2. Inhale through your nose and pull the testicles up. Hold and exhale slowly, lowering your testicles and feeling cool energy in the scrotum. Repeat 9 times.

3. Inhale and pull the energy up to the Sperm Palace, hold, then exhale slowly. Repeat 9 times.

4. Guide the energy up the back as if sipping on a straw. Press the lower back outward as if flattening it against a wall to activate the sacral and cranial pumps. Hold attention on the sacrum and exhale slowly.

5. Relax sacrum and neck.

6. Inhale and guide the energy up to T11, and then relax and exhale.

7. Inhale and guide the energy up to the Jade Pillow at the base of the skull, and then relax and exhale.

8. On the final inhalation, guide the energy up to the crown. At the Crown point, spiral the energy in your brain 9–36 times clockwise, then 9–36 times counterclockwise.

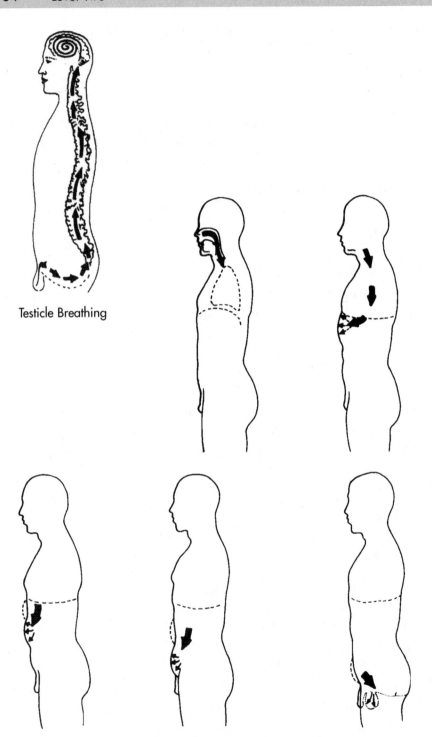

Testicle Breathing

Scrotal Compression

9. After spiraling at the Crown point, place your tongue on your palate and allow the energy to flow down to the third eye, tongue, throat, and heart. Pause for a while at the heart and feel the sexual (creative) energy transform into loving energy, and then move down to the solar plexus and the navel. Collect the energy at the navel.

Scrotal Compression
(Pages 75–77)

1. Sit on the edge of a chair with testicles hanging loose over the edge.
2. Inhale deeply, expanding the solar plexus, while contracting the anus and pulling energy into the upper abdomen.
3. Compress the energy into a sphere at the solar plexus point. Roll this chi ball down the front of the abdomen to the navel, and then down to the pelvic region.
4. Contract the abdominal muscles downward and pack and compress chi into the scrotum for as long as you can. Squeeze the anus and tighten the perineum to prevent energy loss.
5. While maintaining the compression, keep your tongue pressed against your palate to maintain energy flow in the Microcosmic Orbit. Swallow deeply into the sexual center.
6. Exhale. Take a few quick short breaths by pulling your lower abdomen in and pushing it out (Bellows Breathing) until you can breathe normally. Relax completely.
7. Repeat the exercise from 3–9 times until you feel the testicles become warm.
8. Collect energy at the navel and do Bone Breathing.

BONE MARROW NEI KUNG

⟳ Sexual Power Lock Practice (Male)

(Pages 70–75)

1. Sit with your feet flat on the floor. Stimulate your jade staff and direct the sexual energy to your testicles and prostate.

2. When you are near or in the midst of an orgasm, inhale deeply through the nose. At the same time, clench your jaw and both fists, claw your feet, tighten the cranial pump at the back of your neck, and press your tongue firmly to the roof of your mouth.

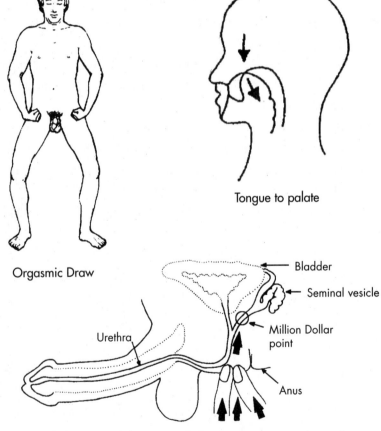

Tongue to palate

Orgasmic Draw

Bladder

Seminal vesicle

Urethra

Million Dollar point

Anus

The Sexual Power Lock for men includes pressing against the urethra with three fingers from a point at the back of the perineum, which puts pressure on the Million Dollar point.

3. Inhale again, drawing up the entire anus and genital region— especially the front part of the perineum. Hold breath then inhale again. Hold breath again while you contract and pull down the front part of the anus, pulling energy to collect at the perineum.

4. Inhale without exhaling, then clench and pull up your sexual region 9 times, holding energy at the front part of the perineum. Exhale and release all the muscles of the body.

5. Repeat steps 1–3 again, this time continuing to pull the energy up through the perineum and into the coccyx and sacrum. Contract the middle and back parts of the anus as you do this. Arch your sacrum back and outward to activate the sacral pump. Hold the energy here and inhale 3–9 times, creating contractions to pull the energy from the sexual organs. Then exhale and relax.

6. Repeat steps 1–3 again, now drawing the sexual energy up through the perineum and sacrum to T11. Hold the energy at T11, then add the energy from the Sperm Palace by inhaling and contracting 9 times without exhaling. Then exhale and relax, mentally guiding energy from the Sperm Palace to T11.

7. Repeat steps 1–3 again, drawing the energy all the way up to C7. At C7, push the top of the sternum back toward the spine to increase the pumping of energy and to activate the thymus.

8. Repeat the same steps again, this time drawing energy to the Jade Pillow. To activate the cranial pump there, tuck the chin in. Clench your teeth, squeeze the back of your skull, and press your tongue hard against your palate to increase the pumping action.

9. Repeat again, now drawing energy to the Crown point, Pai Hui. Turn your eyes and all senses to the top of the skull and press your tongue firmly to your palate. Practice 9 hard contractions and continue to inhale, each time pulling energy from the Sperm Palace to the crown. With your mind, eyes, and senses, spiral the energy at the crown 9–36 times clockwise, then counterclockwise.

10. Rest and allow the energy to enter your brain. Let extra energy run down the Functional Channel to the mid-eyebrow point, nose, throat, heart center, solar plexus, and navel.

BONE MARROW NEI KUNG

🌀 Male Sexual Energy Massage

(Pages 65–88)

🌸 Preliminary Steps

1. Male Power Lock: Inhale 9 short sips of breath as you contract the genital, anal, and perineal areas. Press your tongue against the palate and clench the buttocks and teeth. Use your three middle fingers to press against the back of the perineum to help guide the rising energy up through the sacrum, T11, C7, Jade Pillow, and into the crown.

2. Preliminary cloth massage: Massage genitals, perineum, and sacrum with a silk cloth. Rotate the cloth around the genitals 36 times clockwise, then 36 times counterclockwise. Feel the testicles loose and full of chi.

🌸 The Massage

Rub your hands together briskly to warm them up before performing each of the following steps.

3. Finger massaging the testicles: Inhale chi into testicles, and hold one testicle in each hand, with thumbs on top and the fingers underneath. Gently press your thumbs on each testicle, then use the thumbs to massage the whole testicle: 36 times in clockwise circles, then 36 times in counterclockwise circles. Use your fingers to roll the testicles against your thumbs. Roll them back and forth 36 times.

4. Palm massage: Warm your hands, then cup your testicles in your left hand while moving your penis aside with the back of the right hand. Lightly press the testicles with both palms, then gently rub them with the left palm—36 times clockwise and 36 times counterclockwise. Warm your hands again, then reverse hand positions and massage with the right palm 36 times in each direction. Draw the energy upward.

5. Duct elongation rub: Warm your hands, then cup one testicle in each hand. Use your thumbs and index fingers to gently massage the ducts.

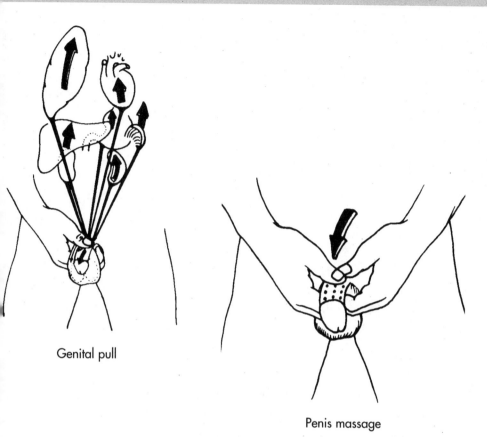

Genital pull

Penis massage

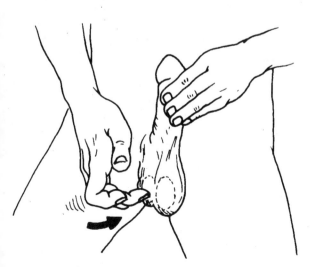

Testicle tapping

Start at the base of the testicles, rubbing the ducts toward the back and the front. Work your way along the ducts toward the body, then reverse direction. Draw energy into the Microcosmic Orbit.

6. Duct-stretching massage: Hold the ducts between your thumbs and index fingers. Gently rub your thumbs toward the center, and use your index fingers to lightly pull the testicles out, stretching the ducts. Repeat 36 times, palm-massaging the testicles in between rounds. Draw the energy upward.

7. Scrotum and penis tendon stretch: Warm your hands, then encircle the base of the penis with your thumb and forefinger while your other fingers surround the testicles. Gradually pull the genitals down as you pull the internal organs up, stretching the whole groin. Next pull the genitals down toward the left as you pull up the internal organs. Hold awhile then release, then pull the genitals down toward the right while pulling the organs up. Finally, pull the genitals downward in a circular motion 9–36 times clockwise, then counterclockwise. Draw the energy upward.

8. Penis massage: Use thumbs and index fingers to hold the base of the penis from the sides. Massage the penis along each of three lines, from base to tip and back. Massage each line up and back 36 times.

9. Testicle tapping: Standing in Horse stance, inhale chi into the testicles—pulling them up slightly—and hold your breath. Clench your teeth while contracting the perineum and anus. Lift your penis out of the way with your left hand, and tap the fingertips of your right hand lightly on the right testicle. Tap in sets of 6, 7, or 9. Exhale, rest, and draw energy up the spine, then change hands and repeat with left testicle.

10. Practice the Power Lock, Genital Compression, and the Silk Cloth Massage.

BONE MARROW NEI KUNG

◉ Female Sexual Energy Massage

(Pages 65–75, 89–94)

❀ Preliminary Steps

1. Female Power Lock: Inhale 9 short sips of breath as you contract the genital, anal, and perineal areas. Press your tongue against the palate and clench the buttocks and teeth. Use your three middle fingers to press against the back of the perineum to help guide the rising energy up through the sacrum, T11, C7, Jade Pillow, and into the crown.

2. Preliminary cloth massage: Massage the vaginal muscles, perineum, coccyx, and sacrum with a silk cloth. Spiral at each location 36 times clockwise and 36 times counterclockwise. Feel enlarged breasts and moist vagina.

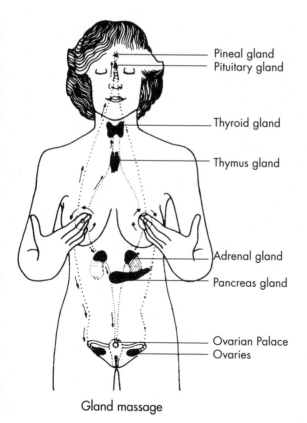

Pineal gland
Pituitary gland

Thyroid gland

Thymus gland

Adrenal gland

Pancreas gland

Ovarian Palace
Ovaries

Gland massage

Activate the endocrine glands by massaging the area around the nipples, using the three middle fingers of each hand.

✿ The Massage

Rub your hands together briskly to warm them up before performing each of the following steps.

3. Breast massage: Sit naked or loosely clothed, with some pressure on the vagina. Pull up the middle and back parts of the anus, drawing the chi up the spinal cord. Pull up the left and right sides of the anus, bringing the chi into the left and right nipples. Warm your hands by rubbing them briskly together, then place the second joint of the middle fingers on the nipples. Place the tongue on the roof of your mouth.

4. Gland massage: Place three fingers on each breast and circle outward from the nipples—clockwise for the right hand and counterclockwise for the left hand. Then circle inward. Repeat the outward and inward circles with the right hand moving counterclockwise and the left hand moving clockwise.

5. Continue massaging as you bring attention to the pituitary gland—the mid-eyebrow point—and then back to the breasts. Draw activated energy into the thyroid and parathyroid glands, then back to the breasts. Continue to gently massage the breasts and focus on the thymus gland, then the breasts, then the pancreas, then back to the breasts. Activate the adrenal glands, then bring this energy up to the breasts to join with the other energies there.

6. Organ massage: Warm your hands and place them on your breasts. Let the chi from the thymus and the breasts activate the chi of the lungs, then return that chi to the breasts. Direct the accumulated chi to activate the heart, then return it to the breasts, and repeat this process with the spleen, kidneys, and liver. Then place your palms on your knees and focus attention on your breasts, letting energy expand into the nipples.

7. Let the accumulated energy in the nipples flow down into the ovaries. Breathe directly into the ovaries as you contract the labia in short pulses, then pull the labia in. Merge energy from both ovaries in the

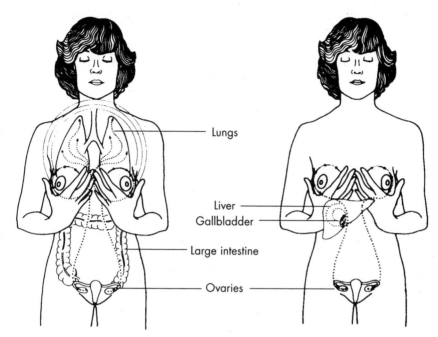

Chi of the lungs and large intestines	Liver and gallbladder chi

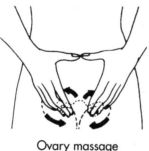

Ovary massage

Ovarian Palace—3 inches below the navel. Tense the cervix and concentrate sexual energy in the Ovarian Palace.

8. Ovary massage: Place your fingertips on your ovaries and massage them in small circles—36 times clockwise and 36 times counterclockwise.

9. Practice the Power Lock, Genital Compression, and the silk cloth massage.

10. If you wish, you can do the Egg Exercise at this point (see page 65 in this book or *Bone Marrow Nei Kung,* pages 94–100).

BONE MARROW NEI KUNG

Male Chi Weight Lifting

(Pages 146–52)

1. Do chi pressure and kidney pressure exercises (see pages 46–49 in level one). Do Male Sexual Energy Massage and the Power Lock 2–3 times).

2. Fold cloth to 1 inch width. Hold it beneath the perineum and bring it behind the testicles. Keeping the cloth edge folded away from the skin, wrap both ends upward around the penis and testicles. Tie a knot at the base of the penis near the pubic bone.

3. Move the knot behind the testicles and beneath the perineum. Let the ends of the cloth hang to the floor. Contract the perineal muscles and tighten the knot. The penis and testicles will bulge slightly.

4. Tie one end of the cloth to the weight as it rests on a chair or the floor.

5. Slowly assume lift stance (feet shoulder-width apart, knees slightly bent) holding the cloth or weight in hand. Test weight with your fingers.

6. Inhale a sip of air and pull up the anus, perineum, and genitals. Inhale again a pull up both sides of the anus, drawing chi into the left and right kidneys.

7. Press tongue to the palate and slowly release cloth. Test the weight gradually and be sure you are not too uncomfortable.

8. Inhale and pull up the right, left, front, and back sides of the anus and wrap energy around the kidneys.

9. Inhale as you contract the anus and perineum and gently swing the weight, drawing energy up to the coccyx and the sacrum. Inhale with each forward swing and exhale with the backward swings.

10. With each inhalation/forward swing, pull up against the weight internally and draw the energy up through the Microcosmic Orbit.

11. Swing the weight 36–49 times for the first week or so, then try 60 times; each swing (forward and back together) should last approximately 1 second.

12. Press your tongue to your palate and bring the energy down to your navel. Advanced students may practice another round, this time lifting the weight from the internal organs and glands.

13. Remove the weight, then finish with 2–3 rounds of the Power Lock followed by Sexual Energy Massage and silk cloth massage. Rest, then practice the Microcosmic Orbit.

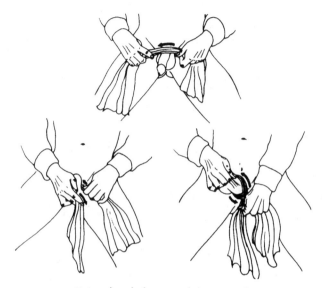

Tying the cloth around the genitals

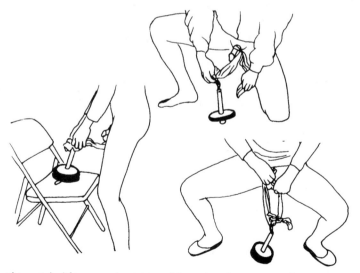

Chi weight lifting can be initiated from kneeling or standing position.

BONE MARROW NEI KUNG

Female Chi Weight Lifting

(Pages 153–62)

1. Do the Egg Exercise as preparation. Pass the string through the egg and knot it at the large end. Tie the weight to the other end of the string.

2. Practice Female Sexual Energy Massage and the Power Lock (3 times).

3. Kneel near the weight and insert the egg's large end into the vagina. Close your vagina, contracting muscles around the egg to hold it.

4. Slowly assume lift stance (feet shoulder-width apart, knees slightly bent), holding the string or weight in hand. Test weight with your fingers.

5. Inhale a sip of air and pull up the anus, perineum, and genitals. Inhale again and pull up both sides of the anus, drawing chi into the left and right kidneys.

6. Press tongue to the palate and slowly release cloth. Test the weight gradually and be sure you are not too uncomfortable.

7. Inhale and pull up the right, left, front, and back sides of the anus and wrap energy around the kidneys.

8. Inhale as you contract the anus and perineum and gently swing the weight, drawing energy up to the coccyx and the sacrum. Inhale with each forward swing and exhale with the backward swings.

9. With each inhalation/forward swing, pull up against the weight internally and draw the energy up through stations of the Microcosmic Orbit.

10. Swing the weight 36–49 times for the first week or so, then try 60 times; each swing (forward and back together) should last approximately 1 second.

11. Press your tongue to your palate and bring the energy down to your navel. Advanced students may practice another round, this time lifting the weight from the internal organs and glands.

12. Remove the weight, then finish with 2–3 rounds of the Power Lock followed by Sexual Energy Massage and silk cloth massage. Rest, then practice the Microcosmic Orbit.

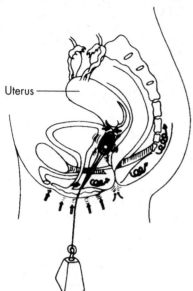

Uterus

Vaginal Weight Lifting

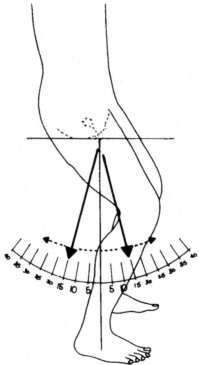

Swing the weight at an angle
between 15 and 30 degrees.

FUSION OF THE FIVE ELEMENTS

Formula 1: Forming Four Pakuas and the Pearl

(Pages 23–35)

1. Sit up straight with your eyes closed and your tongue touching your palate. Do the Inner Smile meditation.
2. Form the front pakua: Turn your awareness and senses in toward the navel. Blend and condense all the energies you have generated into an energy ball at the navel.
3. Beginning at a point 1.5 inches inside the navel and a little above it, draw with your mind the first line of the pakua's outer layer. Continue drawing the other seven lines of the outer layer.
4. Draw the middle layer, one line at a time, and the inner layer one line at a time.
5. Draw eight spokes from the outer layer to the inner one, allowing the spokes to continue into the Tai Chi symbol in the middle. Spiral the Tai Chi symbol clockwise as it blends and transforms the energy. See the pakua glowing with white light, then rest and feel this light.
6. **The back pakua:** Beginning at a point 1.5 inches inside and a little above the Door of Life, trace the outer layer of the pakua line by

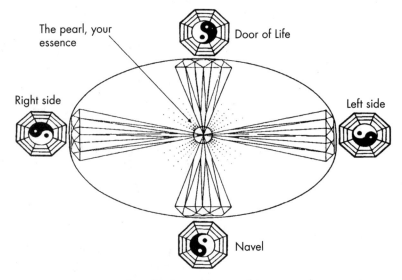

Spiraling the four pakuas to form a pearl

line. Repeat steps 4 and 5 above to complete the back pakua.

7. Spiral the front and back pakuas, especially their Tai Chi centers. Notice the force of the pakuas being drawn through their funnel-like backs toward the cauldron at the center of your body. Focus on the cauldron and draw the energy in. Condense it, and stop spiraling. Let the energy glow with a white light.

8. **The right side pakua:** Focus on the point on the right side of the body that is level with the navel and in line with the armpit, about 1.5 inches inside the body. Draw the outer layer of this pakua, then the middle layer, and then the inner layer. Draw the eight spokes into the center Tai Chi symbol. Spiral this symbol as it fills with light.

9. **The left side pakua:** Focus on the point 1.5 inches inside the left side of the body, at the level of the navel and in line with the left armpit. Draw the three layers line by line, from outside to inside, and draw the spokes. Spiral the Tai Chi symbol at the center.

10. Spiral the centers of the left and right pakuas, drawing their energy through the funnel-like backs and into the cauldron. Join this energy with the energy of the front and back pakuas.

11. **The pearl:** In a relaxed manner, continue spiraling into the cauldron. Bring all your senses down into the cauldron and form the pearl by condensing the essence of all of your life-force energy—the essence of your organs, glands, senses, and mind. Feel the pearl becoming stronger and brighter. Anchor and ground yourself with the pearl using positive affirmations.

12. Move the pearl into the Microcosmic Orbit, becoming aware of three sources of energy: the universal force (North Star and Dipper) coming in through your crown; cosmic particle force coming in through your mid-eyebrow point; and earth force, supplied at the perineum through the soles of the feet. Move the pearl through the Microcosmic Orbit concentrating on each point: the perineum, coccyx, Door of Life, T11, C7, Jade Pillow, crown, mid-eyebrow, throat, heart, solar plexus, and navel.

13. If the pearl diminishes at any time, form a new one by concentrating on the four pakuas and condensing the energy into a pearl.

14. Collect energy at the navel and finish with Chi Self-Massage.

☯ Formula 2: Balancing Your Inner Climate

(Pages 36–51)

1. Sit up with your eyes closed and practice the Inner Smile meditation.
2. Form the front pakua and become aware of the kidneys, making the kidneys' sound, choo-oo-oo-oo. Contract the left and right sides of the anus and pack the kidneys. Form a sphere at the perineum—the kidneys' collection point—by inhaling, pulling up the perineum, and pushing the lower abdomen down toward the perineum. Mentally form a sphere and let it glow with a blue color. Spiral the energy in both kidneys into their collection point. Intensify the spiral there, feeling a force drawing in the kidney's cold energy.
3. Become aware of the heart and thymus gland. Inhale and pull the anus up toward the heart, then pack the heart. Mentally form a sphere at the sternum, the heart's collection point, and let it glow with a red color. Make the heart's sound, haw-w-w-w-w-w, and spiral the energy at the heart, thymus, and the collection point. Allow the spiral at the collection point to draw in the hot energy of the heart and thymus.

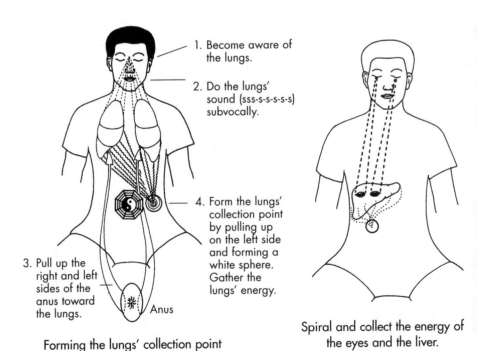

1. Become aware of the lungs.

2. Do the lungs' sound (sss-s-s-s-s) subvocally.

4. Form the lungs' collection point by pulling up on the left side and forming a white sphere. Gather the lungs' energy.

3. Pull up the right and left sides of the anus toward the lungs.

Anus

Forming the lungs' collection point

Spiral and collect the energy of the eyes and the liver.

4. Divide your attention between the cold energy of the kidneys and the hot energy of the heart. Spiral the collection points and the front pakua, then increase the spiral of the front pakua, even spiraling your body a bit to increase the force. Let this pakua draw in the energy from the heart and kidney collection points, blending the cold kidney energy with the hot heart energy.

5. Adapt steps 2–4 to blend the liver and lung energies in the front pakua: focus on the liver and make the liver's sound, sh-h-h-h-h-h. Inhale and contract the right side of the anus toward the liver, then contract the liver. Form the liver/gallbladder collection point under the right side of the ribcage at the level of the navel and in line with the nipple. Form a bright green 3-inch sphere by inhaling and pulling up the right side of the anus as you push down the right side of your body. Spiral the energies of the liver and gallbladder as you spiral this collection point, allowing the sphere to draw in the moist warm energy of the liver and gallbladder.

6. Form the lung/large intestine collection point on the left side of the body, under the left nipple at the level of the navel: Make the lungs' sound, sss-s-s-s-s-s, then inhale as you pull up the left and right sides of the anus toward the lungs. Contract the lungs, then inhale again as you pull up the anus to the level of the navel. Picture the 3-inch metallic white sphere that is the collection point for the lungs and large intestine. Spiral and draw the cool, dry energy of the lungs into this collection point.

7. Divide your attention between the warm, moist energy of the liver and the cool, dry energy of the lungs. Spiral them both, then spiral the front pakua until it is strong enough to draw in the liver and lung energies. Blend them together in the front pakua until the energy there is neither too warm nor too cool, not too wet or too dry.

8. Draw the spleen's energy into the front pakua: Make the spleen's sound, who-o-o-o-o-o, then inhale and pull up the left side of the anus toward the spleen. Contract the back muscles lightly to feel the spleen, then form the spleen's collection point (yellow) at the center of the front pakua. Spiral the energy of the spleen and the front pakua, drawing the spleen's mild energy into the pakua.

9. Repeat steps 2–8 for the back pakua, collecting any remaining organ energies at the secondary collection points that follow. For the kidneys, make a sphere at the sacrum; for the heart, make a sphere behind the heart between T5 and T6. Spiral and blend the hot and cold energies in the back pakua. Collect remaining liver energies at the point to the right rear of the back pakua, and lung energies at the left rear of the back pakua. Spiral and blend the moist and dry energies of the liver and lungs in the back pakua.

10. Spiral the energies of the front and back pakuas, then condense them and draw them into the cauldron. Blend.

11. Form the right side pakua and collect energies from the right side collection points, then do the same for the left side pakua. (See *Fusion of the Five Elements,* pages 47–49, for the locations of these collection points.) Pull the energies from the right and left pakuas into the cauldron, and blend them with the energy there.

12. Condense the blended energy in the cauldron into a refined pearl, then anchor your feelings of peace and harmony to this pearl. Bring the pearl down to the perineum and circulate it in the Microcosmic Orbit, acknowledging the universal, cosmic particle, and earth forces as they are drawn to the pearl.

13. Collect energy at the navel, then practice Chi Self-Massage.

Formula 3: Connecting the Senses
(Pages 52–63)

1. **Ears/Kidneys:** Practice the Inner Smile meditation, then massage your ears and kidneys. Concentrate on the ears by spiraling the energy there, then spiral the energy at the kidneys until it is strong enough to draw in the energy from the ears. Collect the sense of hearing and the kidneys' cold energy in the kidneys. Create a blue sphere at the perineum (the kidneys' collection point) and spiral the energy there to draw in both the hearing energy of the ears and the cold energy of the kidneys.

2. **Tongue/heart:** Move your tongue to generate saliva, and gently massage the heart. Spiral energy at the tongue, and swallow saliva as you spiral the tongue's essence toward the heart. Spiral heart energy to draw

in the tasting energy of the tongue. Make a red sphere at the heart's collection point (sternum), and create a strong spiral there. Draw in both the energy of tasting and the hot red energy of the heart.

3. Spiral the energies of the two collection point into the front pakua, and blend them. Notice the senses being pulled within.

4. **Eyes/liver:** Move your eyes and massage the eyes and liver. Spiral the energy at the eyes, and make a stronger spiral at the liver, drawing the seeing energy of the eyes into the liver. Create a green sphere at the collection point below the liver (in line with the nipple at the level of the navel). Spiral and collect the warm, moist energy of the liver and the energy of sight.

5. **Nose/lungs:** Massage the nose and lungs. Spiral energy in both places, using the stronger spiral at the lungs to draw in the smelling energy of the nose. Make a white sphere at the collection point below the lungs, and spiral the energy there. Draw in the cool, dry energy of the lungs and the essence of the sense of smell.

6. Spiral at the front pakua, drawing in and blending the energies of the eyes and liver with those of the nose and lungs. Feel the senses drawing in and focusing.

7. **Mouth/spleen:** Move your lips and massage the spleen. Spiral the energies in both places, allowing the strong spiral at the spleen to draw in the energy of the mouth. Form a collection point (yellow sphere) in the center of the front pakua and draw in the energies of the spleen and the mouth.

8. Focus your awareness on the back pakua, its collection points, and the energies it has gathered. Spiral the front and back pakuas into the cauldron and blend their energies there. Then do the same for the left and right pakuas, spiraling their energies together into the cauldron. Feel the senses under one center of control. Form a pearl, and anchor your feelings of self-control to it with affirmations. Then bring the pearl to the perineum and circulate it in the Microcosmic Orbit, noticing the universal, cosmic particle, and earth forces that are supplying you. Bring the pearl back to the cauldron and collect energy at the navel. End with Chi Self-Massage.

✿ Formula 4: Transforming Emotions

(Pages 64–81)

1. In a sitting position, practice the Inner Smile meditation. When ready, form the front pakua.

2. **Kidneys/ears:** Turn your attention toward your ears and your kidneys. Become aware of fear, along with any other unpleasant sensations. (These energies may manifest as chilliness, murky blue color, awkward shapes, etc.) Spiral the fear and other sensations out of the kidneys to the kidneys' collection point.

3. **Heart/tongue:** Bring your awareness to your tongue and your heart. Become aware of any feelings of impatience, cruelty, or other unpleasant sensations, which may manifest as feelings, shapes, sounds, or images. Negative feelings of the heart can be perceived as a muddy red color, acidity, heat, and/or noise. Spiral and breathe the emotions and sensations out of the heart, drawing them into the heart's collection point.

4. Spiral these energies from the kidney and heart collection points into the front pakua. Blend them and allow them to transform into a pure

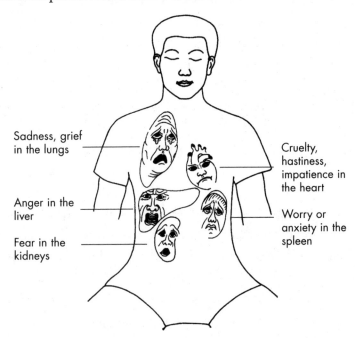

Negative emotions and the organs

energy that is bright and golden. This energy radiates love, joy, and gentleness from your center.

5. **Liver/eyes:** Move your eyes and become aware of your liver. Notice any feelings of anger or other unpleasant sensations. These may be perceived as a steamy or expanding feeling, a murky green or red rage, or a sense of destructiveness. Spiral the anger and any other energies you do not like into the liver's collection point.

6. **Lungs/nose:** Inhale and exhale, then inhale again. Become aware of the connection between the lungs and the nose. Recognize any feelings of sadness, grief, or depression. Negative energy in the lungs can be gray, cold, musty, or salty. Spiral and breathe out the sadness and any other energies you do not want into the lungs' collection point.

7. Spiral the energies from the liver and lung collection points into the front pakua. Blend and balance them, helping them transform to the golden light of kindness and courage.

8. Bring awareness to your mouth and spleen, becoming aware of feelings of worry and anxiety. Negative energy of the spleen can be perceived as cloudy, sour, shaky, uncertain, or sticky. Spiral and breathe the worry and other unpleasant sensations into the spleen's collection point. Bring it to the front pakua to blend with the energies already there.

9. Revisit each of the organs and their collection points, spiraling and drawing out any remaining negative energy and blending it with the other energy in the front pakua. Spiral, blend, and transform all remaining energy, feeling the positive virtues grow. Draw on the love and joy in the heart if you need more resources.

10. Form the back pakua and become aware of all of the energies you have collected there. Spiral the front and back pakuas to draw their energies into the cauldron. Then create and spiral the left and right pakuas to draw their energies into the cauldron. Fuse and condense the energies from all four pakuas in the cauldron and form a pearl, which now glows a brilliant golden color.

11. Bring the pearl down to the perineum and circulate it in the Microcosmic Orbit, feeling the univeral, cosmic particle, and earth forces that supply you. Collect energy at the navel and practice Chi Self-Massage.

🌀 Formula 5: Birth of the Immortal Fetus
(Pages 82–101)

1. Practice Fusion formulas 1–4, fusing the energies from the combined practices in the cauldron and forming a brilliant golden pearl. Bring the pearl down to the perineum and circulate it in the Microcosmic Orbit, maintaining awareness of the universal, cosmic particle, and earth forces supplied to you. Build up the momentum of the pearl.

2. Activate the cranial pump by pressing the tip of your tongue against your lower teeth and the flat of the tongue against the palate. Clench teeth, tilt chin in, pull the eyes in, and turn the ears, nose, and tongue toward the back of the head as you turn all the senses up toward the crown. Feel the pulsations of the cranial pump.

3. Activate the sacral pump by inhaling, pulling up the perineum, then inhaling again as you pull up the back of the anus toward the sacrum. Inhale more, and pull the pearl from the perineum to the sacrum, up to T11, C7, the base of the skull, and the crown. Inhale and hold, feeling a shiny wave of light emerging from the crown.

4. Inhale and swallow your saliva. Feel the crown open. Swallow saliva upward and feel a push up to the crown. Exhale forcefully toward the crown and shoot the pearl out, to a point approximately 6 inches (15.24 centimeters) above the head.

5. Use your senses to control the pearl, learning to move it up, down, and in all directions. Learn to spiral it to the left and right, fast and slow, etc. Then raise it 1 foot higher and practice controlling it again. Continue to raise and control in 1-foot increments until you reach a height that is equal to the height of your body.

🌸 Advanced Fusion Practices
(Pages 91–101)

6. Relax your mind and senses, and use them to to expand the pearl. Shape it into a form similar to your own body, or an idealized/sacralized body—with a head, arms, hands, legs, feet, etc. Then use your senses to

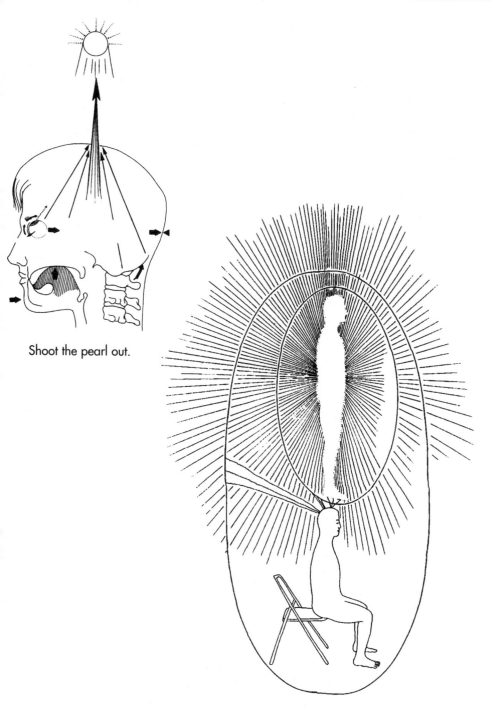

Shoot the pearl out.

Forming an energy body, its protective shield,
and a great bubble to protect all

"carve" the face. Begin by focusing your awareness on your own eyes, then condense their essence into a ball. Activate the crown and exhale the ball of eye energy through it to the face of the energy body. Position the eyes on the energy body's face and affirm that they have been formed. Repeat these steps to place the ears, nose, mouth, and tongue on the energy body.

7. You can alter the face and body's proportions to suit your liking at this time. Then copy the cauldron from your physical body to your energy body: Concentrate on the cauldron and condense it, then shoot it up through your crown into the perineum of the energy body.

8. Assign a gender to your energy body. When this energy being is sharply defined, give it an inner name (which must not be shared with others, for your protection) and an inner voice—or several voices. As your practice develops, these voices will be able advise you.

9. In your physical body, form another pearl in the cauldron and circulate it in the Microcosmic Orbit. Inhale, activate the cranial and sacral pumps, and activate the lead light. Aim the lead light at the perineum of the energy body and shoot the pearl through the crown of your physical body and into the energy body. Use your senses to move the pearl to the sacrum of the energy body, and let it develop there. Then circulate the pearl through the Microcosmic Orbit of the energy body: Door of Life, T11, C7, base of the skull, crown, mid-eyebrow point, tongue, throat, heart, solar plexus, navel, sexual center, and perineum.

10. Form another pearl in your physical body and circulate it in the Microcosmic Orbit to gain momentum. Then return the pearl to the perineum, inhale, and activate the cranial pump. Contract the perineum, anus, and the back of the anus, then pull the pearl up as follows: to the sacrum, Door of Life, T11, C7, and the base of the skull. Draw the pearl toward the back of the crown to a point 1.5 inches behind the crown. Feel a pulsation here, then exhale and shoot the pearl out. When the pearl leaves the crown, use it to form a bubble around the entire energy body.

11. Repeat step 10, forming another pearl, circulating it, and shooting it out from the crown. When the pearl leaves the crown, use it to form a bubble that encloses both your energy body and your physical body. Maintain awareness of your physical body, your energy body, and the bubbles that form protective shields around them.

12. Finish the practice: Condense the energy body (still within its protective bubble) back into a pearl by drawing energy in through the energy body's navel. Maintain awareness of the energy body's protective shield, and of the larger shield protecting the energy and physical bodies together. Inhale and activate the cranial pump, becoming aware of the lead light at the crown. Inhale and draw the pearl toward the crown, then inhale again with more force to pull the pearl into the body at the crown. Circulate the pearl in the Microcosmic Orbit.

13. Maintaining awareness of the big bubble that surrounds the physical body and the energy body's bubble, inhale and draw the energy body's bubble in through the crown and the back of the crown. Add its energy to the pearl that is circulating. Then begin to shrink the larger protective bubble, by slowly drawing some of it in through the point 1.5 inches behind the crown. Add its energy to the circulating pearl, but keep a portion of the shield around your physical body.

14. Bring the pearl down the front channel to the navel. Draw what remains of your protective shield more tightly around you by pulling it in through the navel. Return the pearl to the cauldron. Spiral and condense your energy at the navel. Practice Chi Self-Massage.

FUSION OF THE FIVE ELEMENTS
☯ Advanced Practice Formulas 6–8

(Pages 102–43)

These practices form the virgin children and their animal offspring, and connect the practitioner with the planetary and earth forces.

1. Practice Fusion formulas 1–4, then fuse the energies from the four pakuas in the cauldron, forming a brilliant golden pearl. Focus attention on your kidneys and their essence of gentleness. Spiral the kidneys' energy to their collection point until it glows with bright blue light. Form the blue light into the image of a pure boy or girl, who epitomizes gentleness. This virgin child is dressed in blue and breathing out a blue breath. The blue breath accumulates and then transforms into a deer with antlers, which embodies the refined pure energy of gentleness. Spiral energy at the kidneys' collection point and exhale through it, projecting an intense wave of gentleness toward the back of your body. This energy will attract the earth force of the north, which can be visualized as a big turtle. Place it at your back to protect your north side, and connect with the planet Mercury.

2. Repeat step 1, focusing this time on the heart, its red color, and its essence of love and joy. Form the red light into a pure boy or girl who is dressed in red and is breathing out a red breath. This red breath transforms into a pheasant, which embodies the pure energy of love and joy. Spiral the force at the heart's collection point, then exhale through it toward the front of your body. This will attract the earth force of the south—fire. Form a pheasant to capture the fire force of the earth, and place it in front of you to protect your south side. Connect above with Mars.

3. Repeat this process again, focusing on the liver, its green color, and its essence of kindness. Form the green light into a pure boy or girl, dressed in green, who is breathing out a green breath—the energy of kindness. Form the breath into a green dragon that epitomizes kindness. Spiral the energy at the liver's collection point and exhale

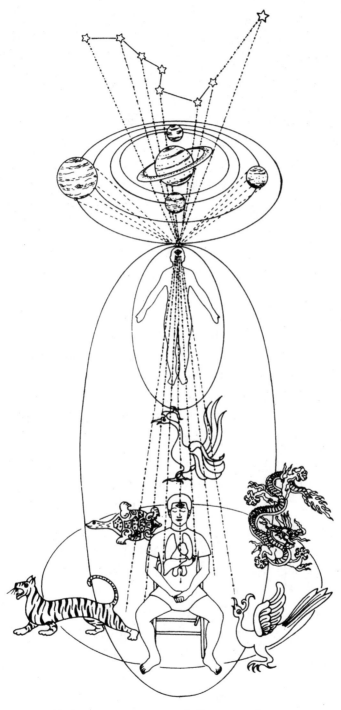

Maintaining awareness of all sources of energy

through it. Form a green dragon—the embodiment of earth's wood force—to the right of your body (east), connecting above with the planet Jupiter.

4. Spiral the lungs' energy to the collection point and form a white light. See the light transform into a virgin child dressed in white who exhales a white breath. This breath transforms into a white tiger—the essence of courage. Spiral energy at the lungs' collection point and exhale through it. The pure energy of the lungs attracts the earth's metal force. Form a white tiger—the embodiment of the earth's metal force—to the left of your body (west), and connect above with Venus.

5. Spiral the spleen's energy to its collection point and form a yellow light. Form the light into a pure child dressed in yellow, who embodies the spleen's virtues of openness and fairness and who exhales a yellow breath. This breath transforms itself into a yellow phoenix—the epitome of fairness. Spiral energy at the spleen's collection point and project it along the centerline of the body out through the top of your head. When this attracts the earth force, form a phoenix, and place it over the top of your head for protection. Connect with Saturn.

6. Form a protective ring around your organs by drawing a circle from the green dragon and virgin child at the liver's collection point up to the virgin child and red phoenix at the heart's collection point. Continue to draw the circle around to the lungs' collection point, down to the kidneys' collection point, and finishing at the center of the front pakua—the spleen's collection point and the place of the yellow phoenix and virgin child.

7. Form a ring of fire around your body connecting the red pheasant, the green dragon, the blue/black turtle, and the white tiger. The yellow phoenix at the top of the body forms a fiery dome.

8. Form a protective bubble and shield as in the previous formula.

9. Collect energy at your navel and finish with Chi Self-Massage.

THE INNER STRUCTURE
OF TAI CHI

🌀 Opening Movements and North Corner,
Left-Hand Form

(Pages 83–92)

1. Stand in Wu Chi stance facing north. Your feet should be together and relaxed and your head pulled up as if suspended from a string. Eyes are open, tongue is touching your palate, and your breathing is even and deep, penetrating to the tan tien.

2. Smile down to your thymus, organs, and navel. Inhale and exhale gently, sinking down from the kua as you exhale: sink your chest to round the scapulae, rotate your palms toward the back, and shift your tailbone over the right heel, shifting weight onto the right leg.

3. When all your weight is on the right leg, inhale and pick up your left heel, sweeping the big toe on the ground as you move your left foot a shoulder-width away from the right foot. Exhale and place your left foot on the ground with all nine points touching. Feel an energy ball at the navel.

4. Inhale, letting your scapulae raise your arms to shoulder height, with elbows pointing downward. Exhale slowly, bending your elbows and sinking the wrists so that the palms face outward. Round the scapulae, tilt your sacrum in, and extend the arms. Exhale and lower the arms with internal chi power, letting the elbows lead until the hands are at the level of the hips.

5. Sink back/First Ward Off: Inhale and sink weight onto the right leg. Allow your tan tien to lead the rotation to the left (west), so that the hips and sacrum turn left. Lift the left toes and pivot the left heel, setting the toes down pointing west. As your waist turns, raise your left hand in a counterclockwise circle to the height of the heart (palm facing downward). Right hand turns palm up and swings to just below the navel, forming a chi ball between the palms.

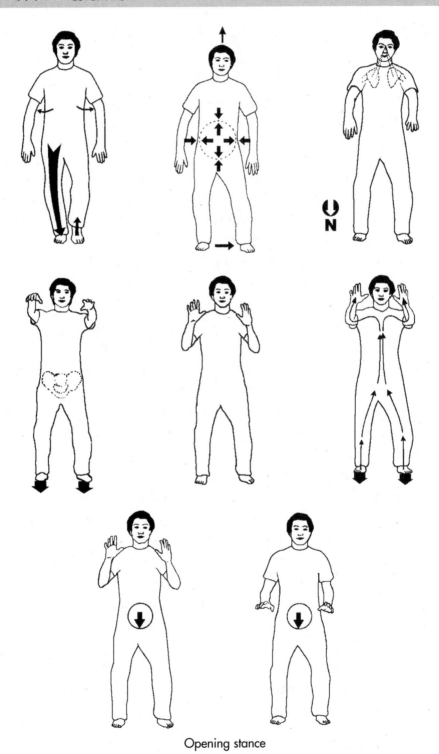

Opening stance

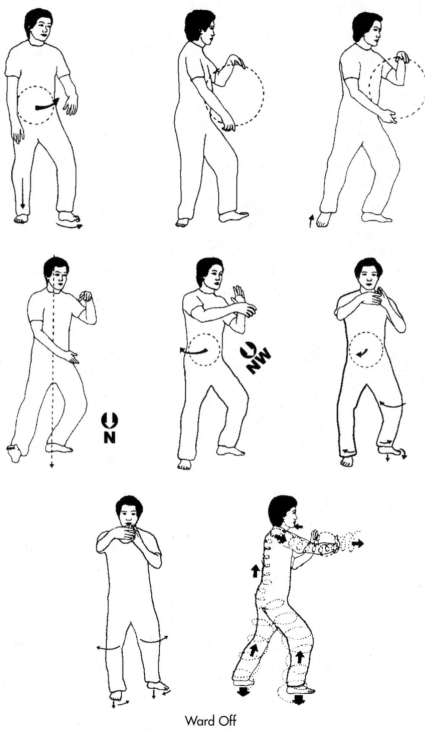

Ward Off

6. Exhale, shifting 60 percent of your body weight to the left foot. Inhale, directing the tan tien energy—which turns the hips—to shift your upper body 45 degrees to the right (northwest). At the same time, shift balance to your left foot and raise the right heel.

7. Second Ward Off: Sink into your left leg and step out wide toward the north with your right foot. Exhale as your foot comes down with the toes pointing directly forward (north). Shift some weight to your right foot as you raise your right arm to the height of your heart, palm facing your chest. Drop your left elbow so your fingers are pointing upward, and the palm faces your right palm. The hands hold an energy ball as the body faces northwest, with the left foot pointing west and the right foot pointing north.

8. Inhale and rotate the left leg inward, turning the foot 45 degrees to face northwest. Let your tan tien turn your hips to the right (north) as the right knee turns outward. Also turn the left leg outward, feeling the earth force transferring energy up the leg. In addition to pushing down and spiraling, the left leg also begins to push forward, allowing the spiraling energy to move upward to the hip and spine.

9. Exhale and shift your weight forward onto the right foot. Use sacral and T11 pumps to propel energy up to C7, then sink the chest, tuck in your chin, and propel the energy like a wave from C7 out through the arms and hands, straightening your right palm.

❂ North Corner, Left-Hand Form (continued)
(Pages 92–96)

10. Rollback: Sink back by inhaling and sinking into the right leg, which pushes into the earth. Bend the left knee, pushing your body back without moving your feet. Straighten your right wrist and point your fingers forward as you rotate your left hand so the palm faces up. Bring the left hand under the right arm to the elbow.

11. Exhale and use your mind to turn your tan tien and waist to the left as the hips torque slightly to the right. Spiral the right arm and rotate your palm toward the face.

12. Press: Inhale as the left arm scoops a circle (palm up). At the same time, the tan tien chi directs the hips to turn back toward the north. At the moment the hips complete their turn to the north, the left hand should complete its circle and come to press on the heel of the right hand. When your hips have turned, exhale and press the left foot to the ground, rotating the knee outward. As the left leg pushes forward, the right knee spirals outward, and spiraling energy moves

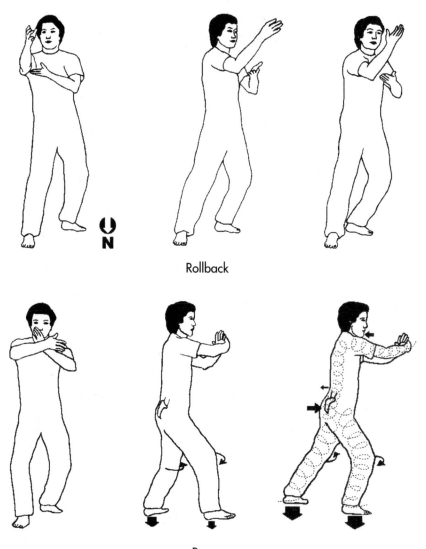

Rollback

Press

up the legs to the sacrum. Activate the sacral pump to bring the energy to T11, and then C7. Sink the chest and round the scapulae to activate the pump at T11 and transfer the force through your arms and hands. As energy reaches your hands, twist the right hand clockwise and the left hand counterclockwise. Pull your chin back to activate the cranial pump.

13. Two-Hand Push: Inhale and sink back onto the left foot. Pull down your sacrum as the heavenly pull stretches the spine up. Your right leg begins to push into the earth, and both palms turn down. Separate the hands to shoulder-width apart. Bring palms to front, forming the Fair Lady's Hand.

14. Press and rotate the legs to drive energy upward as in step 3. Activate the sacral, T11, and C7 pumps to spread energy to the arms, then activate the cranial pump. Let tendon power stretch your fingers as you spiral the left arm/hand clockwise, and the right arm/hand counterclockwise.

15. Single Whip to the south: Sink back into your left leg and straighten your elbows a bit. Your forearms should be parallel to the ground, palms facing down. Lift your right foot slightly onto its heel.

16. Exhale and turn your chi to the left (west), letting the hips follow. Your upper body should be turned by your hips. Pivot your right

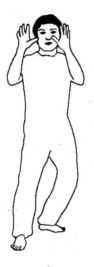
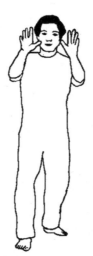
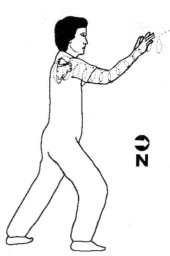

Push

foot on its heel until the toes are also pointing west, then set the foot down. Slowly rotate your spine and upper body to the left until your arms face south. When you've reached your maximum turn to the left, inhale and press your left leg to the ground, shifting your weight onto your right leg. Then exhale as you turn your hips to the right, transferring the coiled energy from your left leg to your right.

17. As you turn your hips, bend your right arm at the elbow and form a beak with the right hand. Simultaneously bring your left hand under your right elbow. Inhale and release the energy coiled in the right leg

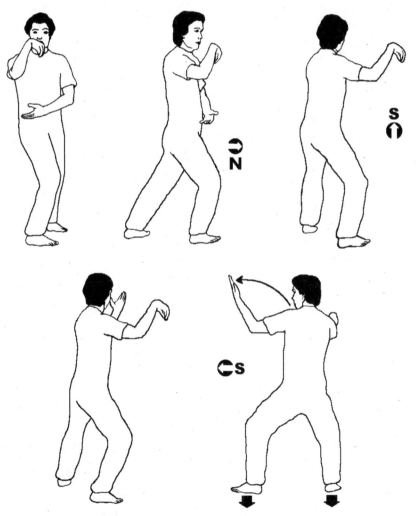

Single Whip

by directing the tan tien chi to turn the hips to the left, and pivoting your left foot on the big toe. The force will travel up the spine through the right arm. Strike beak to the west.

18. Circle Step/Reaching to Heaven: Keeping all of your weight on your right foot (still pointing west), step out wide with your left foot, bringing the heel down 45 degrees to the left of the right heel. Bring down the toes pointing south as you exhale and balance your weight onto both feet. At the same time, the left hand draws an arc about a forearm's length from the face, with the palm facing the body. The left hand opens the palm upward and the right hand retains the beak. The hips are facing southwest.

19. Single-Hand Push: Inhale and pivot the right foot on its heel, turning toes 45 degrees to face southwest. Your mind directs the tan tien chi to turn left, and the hips follow. Exhale and press your right foot into the ground, spiraling energy up the right leg. Turn the hips southward and spiral the energy up into the hips and spine. Activate the sacral, T11, and C7 pumps, transferring the force out through the left arm like a wave. Tuck your chin in to activate the cranial pump.

West, South, and North Corners, Transition to Right-Hand Form

(Pages 101–8)

For the west corner, repeat steps 5–19 from the previous pages, but rotate all directional cues 90 degrees to the left. So if the instruction says toes are pointing west, in this step the toes would be pointing south, and so on.

1. West corner: Begin where the north corner ended, at step 19 above, then sink back onto your right leg and proceed with step 5 above. You are facing west and rotating to the left, which is south.

2. Continue with the Ward Off, Rollback, Press, Push (all to the west), Single Whip (to the east), Circle Step, and Single Hand Push (to the southeast)—steps 6–19.

3. For the south corner, you will repeat steps 5–17 again, ending with

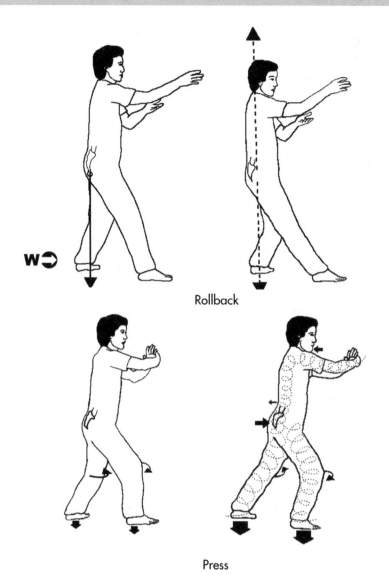

Rollback

Press

a Single Whip to the north. This time you will rotate another 45 degrees to the left, so if the original step says the toes are pointing west, this time the toes will be pointing east. South corner: Ward Off, Rollback, Press, Push, Single Whip.

4. Transition to Right-Hand Form: Facing north, drop both arms to chest level and direct the tan tien chi to turn the hips to the right (northeast). Turn both palms up, as if cradling a baby.

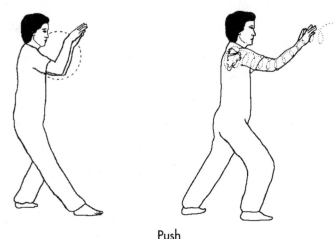

Push
Left-Hand Form: Second Ward Off to west

5. Second Ward Off*: Describe a circle with your right arm, not going above the level of the ear. Shift some weight to your left foot as you raise your left arm to the height of your heart, palm facing your chest. Drop your right elbow so your fingers are pointing upward, and the palm faces your left palm. The hands hold an energy ball as the body faces northeast, with the right foot pointing east and the left foot pointing north.

6. Inhale and rotate the right leg inward, turning the foot 45 degrees to the left. Let your tan tien turn your hips to the left as the left knee turns outward. Also turn the right leg outward, feeling the earth force transferring energy up the leg. In addition to pushing down and spiraling, the right leg also begins to push forward, allowing the spiraling energy to move upward to the hip and spine.

7. Exhale and shift your weight forward onto the left foot. Use sacral and T11 pumps to propel energy up to C7, then sink the chest, tuck in your chin, and propel the energy like a wave from C7 out through the arms and hands, straightening your left palm.

---

*Note that there is no first Ward Off when transitioning to the Right-Hand Form, though subsequent corners will include a first Ward Off. To begin the Right-Hand Form, you will repeat steps 7–19 on pages 116–20, reversing all hand and foot instructions from left to right and vice versa. You will begin facing north and will rotate to the right.

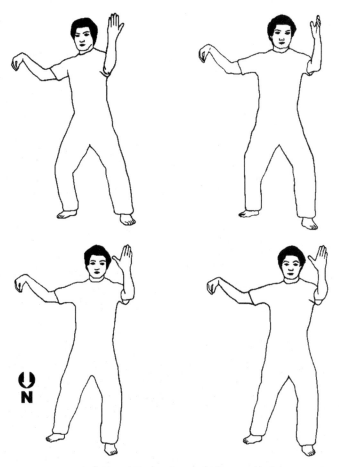

Left-Hand Form: Single Whip to north

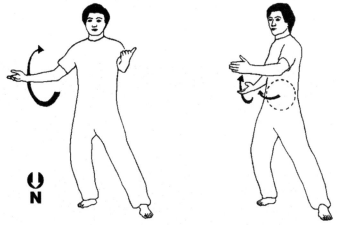

Transition to Right-Hand Form

⚙ North Corner, Right-Hand Form (continued)

(Pages 109–10)

8. Rollback: Sink back by inhaling and sinking into the left leg, which pushes into the earth. Bend the right knee, pushing your body back without moving your feet. Straighten your left wrist and point your fingers forward as you rotate your right hand so the palm faces up. Bring the right hand under the left arm to the elbow.

9. Exhale and use your mind to turn your tan tien and waist to the right as the hips torque slightly to the left. Spiral the left arm and rotate your palm toward the face.

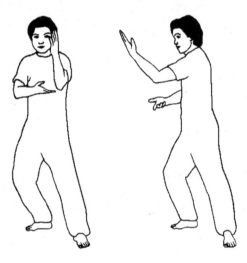

Rollback

10. Press: Inhale as the right arm scoops a circle (palm up). At the same time, the tan tien chi directs the hips to turn back toward the north. At the moment the hips complete their turn to the north, the right hand should complete its circle and come to press on the heel of the left hand. When your hips have turned, exhale and press the right foot to the ground, rotating the knee outward. As the right leg pushes forward, the left knee spirals outward, and spiraling energy moves up

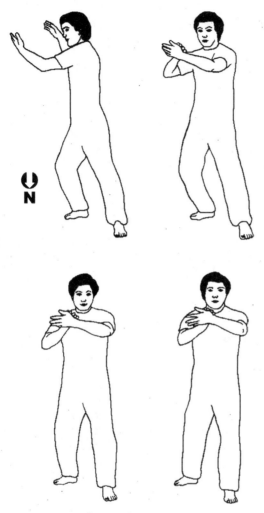

Right-Hand Form: Press to north

the legs to the sacrum. Activate the sacral pump to bring the energy to T11, and then C7. Sink the chest and round the scapulae to activate the pump at T11 and transfer the force through your arms and hands. As energy reaches your hands, twist the left hand clockwise and the right hand counterclockwise. Pull your chin back to activate the cranial pump.

11. Two-Hand Push: Inhale and sink back onto the right foot. Pull down your sacrum as the heavenly pull stretches the spine up. Your left leg begins to push into the earth, and both palms turn down. Separate the hands to shoulder-width apart. Bring palms to front, forming the Fair Lady's Hand.

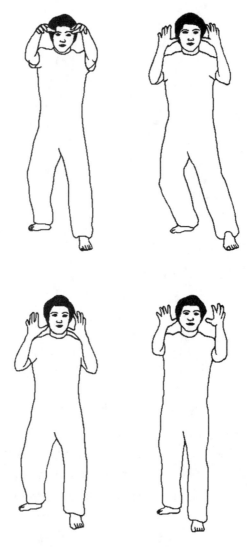

Right-Hand Form: Push to north

12. Press and rotate the legs to drive energy upward as in step 3. Activate the sacral, T11, and C7 pumps to spread energy to the arms, then activate the cranial pump. Let tendon power stretch your fingers as you spiral the right arm/hand clockwise, and the left arm/hand counterclockwise.

13. Single Whip: Sink back into your right leg and straighten your elbows a bit. Your forearms should be parallel to the ground, palms facing down. Lift your left foot slightly onto its heel.

14. Exhale and turn your chi to the right (east), letting the hips follow. Your upper body should be turned by your hips. Pivot your left foot on its heel until the toes are also pointing east, then set the foot down. Slowly rotate your spine and upper body to the right until your arms face south. When you've reached your maximum turn to the right, inhale and press your right leg to the ground, shifting your weight onto your left leg. Then exhale as you turn your hips to the left, transferring the coiled energy from your right leg to your left.

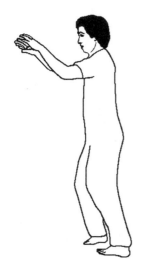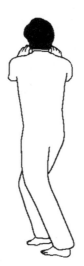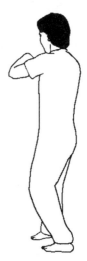

Begin Single Whip

15. As you turn your hips, bend your left arm at the elbow and form a beak with the left hand. Simultaneously bring your right hand under your left elbow. Inhale and release the energy coiled in the left leg by directing the tan tien chi to turn the hips to the right and pivoting your right foot on the big toe. The force will travel up the spine through the left arm. Strike beak to the east.

16. Circle Step/Reaching to Heaven: Keeping all of your weight on your left foot (still pointing east), step out wide with your right foot, bringing the heel down 45 degrees to the right of the left heel. Bring down

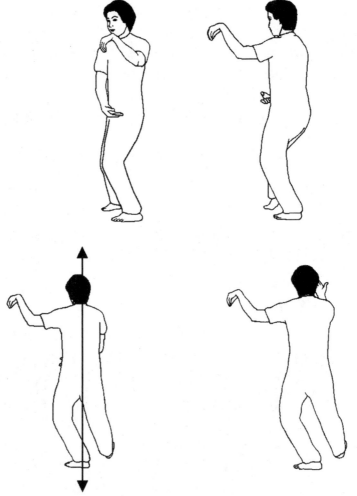

Right-Hand Form: Single Whip to south

the toes pointing south as you exhale and balance your weight onto both feet. At the same time, the right hand draws an arc about a forearm's length from the face, with the palm facing the body. The right hand opens the palm upward and the left hand retains the beak. The hips are facing southeast.

17. Single-Hand Push: Inhale and pivot the left foot on its heel, turning toes 45 degrees to face southeast. Your mind directs the tan tien chi to turn right, and the hips follow. Exhale and press your left foot into the ground, spiraling energy up the left leg. Turn the hips southward and spiral the energy up into the hips and spine. Activate the sacral, T11, and C7 pumps, transferring the force out through the right arm like a wave. Tuck your chin in to activate the cranial pump.

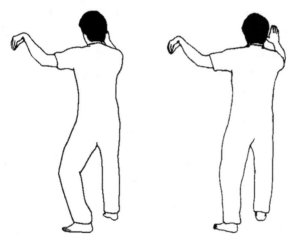

Single-Hand Push

⟳ East and South Corners (Right-Hand Form) to Completion

(Pages 111–18)

1. East corner: Sink back/First Ward Off: Inhale and sink weight onto the left leg. Allow your tan tien to lead the rotation to the right (east), so that the hips and sacrum turn right. Lift the right toes and pivot the right heel, setting the toes down pointing east. As your waist turns, raise your right hand in a counterclockwise circle to the height of the heart (palm facing downward). The left hand turns palm up and swings to just below the navel, forming a chi ball between the palms.

2. Exhale, shifting 60 percent of your body weight to the right foot. Inhale, directing the tan tien energy—which turns the hips—to shift your upper body 45 degrees to the right (northwest). At the same time, shift balance to your right foot and raise the left heel.

3. Repeat steps 6–19 on pages 116–20 above: Ward Off, Rollback, Press, Push, Single Whip, Circle Step, Single-Hand Push.

4. Sink back into your left leg. The right palm drops, facing the chest. Then proceed with the south corner, repeating steps 6–19 above, including Ward Off, Rollback, Press, Push, Single Whip, Circle Step, Single-Hand Push, and sink back.

5. Completion: Inhale and shift your weight onto your left leg. At the same time, raise your hands above your head, palms facing each other. Bring the arms downward in a large circle. Exhale as they pass the level of the shoulders, and simultaneously step straight back with your right foot, touching down a shoulder-width from the left foot, toes facing north. Continue bringing the arms downward as you shift all your weight onto your right leg.

6. Inhale and continue the circular motion of each arm, now bring them up the front of the body so that the wrists cross in front of the navel, with palms facing up. Collect energy through the arms and into the navel. At the same time, step the left foot inward, placing it next to the right foot, with both knees slightly bent. Divide your

weight evenly between the two legs as the hands—still crossed at the wrists—continue to rise in front of the body to the level of the throat.

7. Separate the two hands, palms up, to shoulder-width apart. Then exhale slowly as you turn the palms downward and begin to lower your arms. As the hands approach your waist, slowly straighten your legs, ending the form as you began it—in the Wu Chi stance. Relax and allow all your channels to open. Smile down and collect energy at your navel.

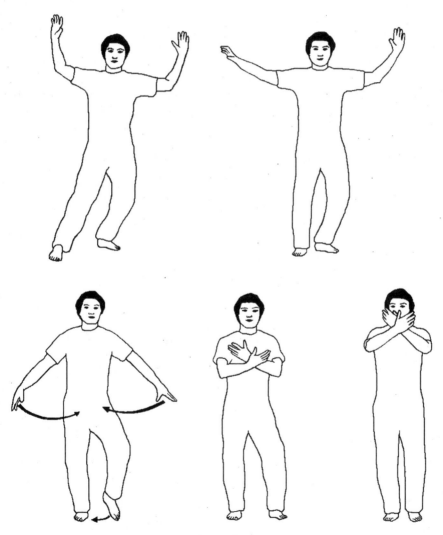

Completing the form

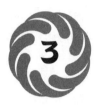

Level Three

The third level of the Universal Healing Tao system consists of more than fifty formulas based on and corresponding to four Destiny Books editions of Universal Healing Tao books: *Taoist Cosmic Healing, Chi Nei Tsang, Cosmic Fusion,* and *The Healing Energy of Shared Consciousness.*

These Level Three practices begin to explore methods of healing the physical and subtle bodies through direct use of chi.

TAOIST COSMIC HEALING

Theory: Cosmic Healing Chi Kung is the cultivation of the ability to conduct chi for the purposes of healing. We call this practice "Cosmic Healing" because we ultimately learn to use the forces of nature, human will, and cosmic particles to transform negativity stored in the body.

Concept: To connect with the energy channels we need to consciously open them in the body. Through the Universal Healing Tao techniques of Bone Marrow Washing, Earth and Heaven Channeling, and Tiger Mouth, among others, we activate our energy lines, channels, and meridians, opening them to our consciousness. With the Cosmic Chi Kung formulas (formally known as Buddha Palm), you can activate the negative and positive channels in the body. These Cosmic Healing techniques will assist you in connecting with your vital organs to grow and experience your internal energy while healing your body.

Purpose: With daily Taoist Cosmic Healing practice, you will open the body's channels to the cosmic forces of heaven and earth, and learn to cultivate them in your body. By growing this cosmic energy and incorporating the elemental and color forces, you will set in motion a total-body healing process.

CHI NEI TSANG

Theory: The ancient Taoists developed the art of Chi Nei Tsang to recycle and transform negative energies that obstruct the internal organs and cause knots in the abdomen. Chi Nei Tsang clears out the toxins, bad emotions, deficient heat, and excessive heat that cause the organs to malfunction. The Chi Nei Tsang formulas are a hands-on application to manually remove stagnation and debris from your energy channels.

Concept: Through the Chi Nei Tsang internal organ massage techniques, the practitioner activates and opens the body channels and energy lines, releasing the sick energy and winds. The Chi Nei Tsang formulas included here detoxify the whole body, removing blockages one at a time. This detoxification may take weeks or months, depending on the extent of the stagnation. Common aliments like headaches and sciatic nerve pain are also addressed.

Purpose: You will learn how to diagnose your body and the bodies of your students, assessing levels of toxicity, obstruction, and stress from the inside out. This is a safe, practical way to connect physically with your body and balance it on a daily basis.

COSMIC FUSION

Theory: The concept of Internal Alchemy is grounded in the Taoist belief that the inner universe is a reflection of the outer universe. There are connections that can be made between the inner and outer universe through which energy—experienced in the inner universe as life force, or chi—can be greatly enhanced by the immense power of the outer universe.

After setting up the energetic composting machine and building the pearl in the Fusion of the Five Elements practices, you need to open up channels of the body with Cosmic Fusion to balance and heal the body.

Concept: Cosmic Fusion practice builds on the foundations of Internal Alchemy that were laid in Fusion of the Five Elements practice. Once the negative emotions have been drawn out and transformed, the pearl is moved through the Creation Cycle, nurturing the virtues. These qualities are cultivated, blended, and condensed into the pearl. The practitioner can now use this highly refined pearl to open and clear four of the eight specific energy channels in the subtle body: the three Thrusting Channels, used for cleansing and protection, and the Belt Channel, the protective belt route that surrounds the Thrusting Channels.

Purpose: During the Fusion practices, the essence of life-force energy found in the organs, glands, and senses is transformed, purified, condensed, and combined with the universal force, the cosmic particle force, and the earth force in order to achieve internal balance. This transformation of quality energy into a harmonious whole can effect positive changes in the human body. Controlling this energy enables each individual to attain balance and harmony of these energies on physical, emotional, and spiritual levels.

HEALING ENERGY OF SHARED CONSCIOUSNESS

Theory: The universe has abundant energy to enhance and multiply the enjoyment of our lives. All that we need to do is connect to the source. These practices teach us to merge the three minds into one mind (Yi) and to employ this unified mind to transform the energy that is directed at us into positive energy. This can result in more balanced, less negative energy for our culture and the institutions created to serve us.

Concept: The World Link of Protection Healing Meditation is a spiritual practice that takes around 15–30 minutes. It offers practitioners access to a method of moving energy—both the energy within them and the energy in their environment—and then focusing it for good intentions and positive transformation. When people from all around the world link together at the same time they are greatly empowered.

Purpose: By linking and synchronizing practice times across the globe, we can create a united world for the manifestation of personal and collective health and healing.

TAOIST COSMIC HEALING
Buddha Palm Opening Practices

(Pages 98–104)

Perform these opening practices before doing any of the core practices that follow. Finish with the closing practices.

Three Minds into One

1. Stand with hands at your sides, armpits open. Empty your mind and heart into your lower tan tien.
2. Hold your hands together at your heart center; smile and feel joy. Extend your hands, legs, and mind deep into the earth and the universe below.
3. Begin Bone Breathing, packing and compressing Universal Chi into your bones.
4. Feeling your tan tien and the universe spiraling, draw this chi into your crown.

Channeling the Earth Force: Marrow Washing

1. Smile into the perineum, palms, and crown. Raise your arms to chest height, palms facing each other. Contract the perineum bridge and the round muscles of the eyes.
2. Expand your mind down to the earth, and feel the Earth Chi being absorbed through your soles into your whole body. Feel it enter the bones and the marrow from your soles to your crown.
3. Tiger Mouth: Raise the index finger on each hand slightly upward, then stretch your thumbs down toward the earth, forming the "tiger's mouth" and activating the Hegu points (LI 4).
4. Slowly lower your hands until the Hegu points (the "eyes" of the hands) are beside the iliac crests (the "eyes" of the hips). Feel your tan tien and crown full with chi, as your tan tien and the universe spiral, activating the lungs and large intestine. Hold for 30 seconds.

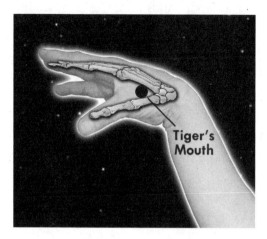

Activating the eye of the hand

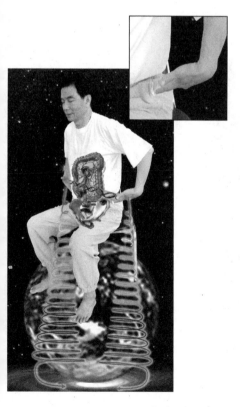
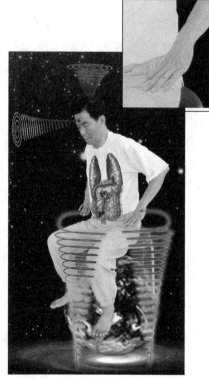

Activating the organ energies

5. Let your Yi rotate your hands until they are palm upward, with the middle fingers pointing toward the eyes of the hips. Feel the tan tien and universe spiraling as you notice the energy flowing back and forth between the tips of your middle fingers via the hip points; this will activate the pericardium.

6. Rotate the fingers forward so that the hip points align with SI 3 on each hand. As the tan tien and universe spiral, let the energy passing from hand to hand activate your heart and small intestine.

🌀 Absorbing the Heavenly Force: Marrow Washing from Crown to Soles

1. Extend your arms forward at chest height, with the palms facing up. Bring your awareness to your tan tien, crown, and your personal star as you expand your Yi to connect to the galaxy. Open the index finger and stretch the thumb forward and down to activate the Laogong point.

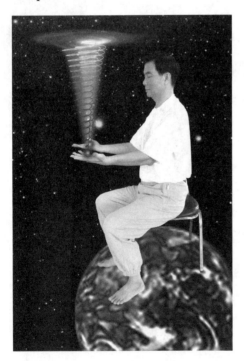

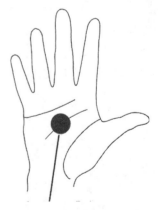

Laogong point
(Pericardium 8)

Draw Heaven Chi into the palms.

2. Feel heavenly energy entering through your palms—the violet light of the North Star and the red light of the Big Dipper. Raise your hands above your head and grasp the handle of the Big Dipper, turning the cup over to pour light over your crown; feel it entering your body through your palms and crown, washing your bones and bone marrow from head to toe. Also be aware of energy bubbling up to your crown through your soles and perineum.

3. Rock your body lightly to keep your spine open.

Absorbing the Earth Force and the Other Side of the Galaxy

1. Bring your arms down to shoulder level, palms facing down.

2. Raise your index fingers slightly and extend the thumbs toward each other and down toward the ground. Focusing most of your attention on the spiraling of your tan tien and the universe, feel the chi enter and fill your fingers and hands, then your arms, then your shoulders, neck, and head. Allow chi to flow from your toes up the legs to your hips, then into your spine and rib cage.

3. Maintaining your awareness of the spiraling tan tien and universe, feel the Laogong points (palms), the Bubbling Spring points (soles), and your perineum activating with earth energy as you smile through the earth to connect with the galaxy and the universe.

4. Draw the combined light of these forces through your palms and soles; let it wash up the center of your bones from your feet upward, steaming and cleansing your marrow. Let any impurities or illness drip from your bones into the earth, where they will be purified and recycled.

TAOIST COSMIC HEALING
Buddha Palm Closing Movements

(Pages 129–34)

Practice these closing movements after any of the core practices. They are performed with your arms extended forward, palms facing downward at the level of the solar plexus. Hold each stage for 5 seconds.

☯ Index fingers

1. Tense all the fingers and feel chi filling all the joints. Open the index fingers by raising them, keeping the other fingers level. Draw Heaven Chi in through the lightly tensed index fingers, and hold for 5 seconds. Relax the hands and bring the index fingers back to neutral position.

2. Stretch and tense the fingers again. This time point the index fingers down to draw in Earth Chi, and circulate it around your body. Hold for 5 seconds, then return the fingers to a neutral position.

3. Once again raise your index fingers to draw in Heaven Chi for 5 seconds, then relax.

☯ Ring fingers

1. Stretch the ring fingers down toward the earth, keeping the other fingers level. Draw Earth Chi in through the ring fingers and circulate it throughout the body, then return your hands to a neutral relaxed position.

2. Stretch the index fingers upward again, drawing in Heaven Chi. Hold for 5 seconds then relax.

☯ Thumbs

1. Stretch your thumbs out and down, drawing Earth Chi in through them. Circulate the Earth Chi in your body, then relax your hands.

2. Stretch your index fingers upward to draw in Heaven Chi. Hold for 5 seconds and relax.

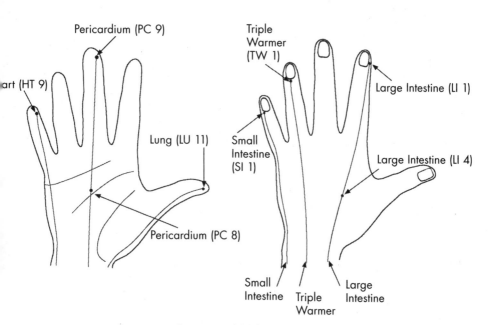

Pericardium (PC 9)

Triple Warmer (TW 1)

art (HT 9)

Large Intestine (LI 1)

Lung (LU 11)

Small Intestine (SI 1)

Large Intestine (LI 4)

Pericardium (PC 8)

Small Intestine

Triple Warmer

Large Intestine

The points of the hand

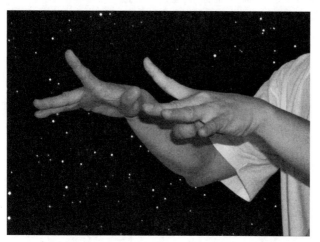

Activate the index fingers to draw in Heaven Chi

Buddha Palm Closing Movements

✪ Pinkie Fingers

1. Stretch your pinkie fingers out and down, drawing Earth Chi in through them. Circulate the Earth Chi in your body, then relax your hands.
2. Stretch your index fingers upward to draw in Heaven Chi. Hold for 5 seconds and relax.

✪ Middle Fingers

1. Stretch your middle fingers out and down, drawing Earth Chi in. Circulate the Earth Chi in your body, then relax your hands.
2. Stretch your index fingers upward to draw in Heaven Chi. Hold for 5 seconds and relax.

✪ Closing Movements: Crane's Beak and Swallow the Saliva

1. Form beaks with both hands by squeezing all of your fingers around the thumbs. Inhale and contract your sexual organs.
2. Move your tongue around and draw in your cheeks to generate saliva; divide the saliva into three parts. Gulp the first part of your saliva down to the center of your navel, the second part down to the left side of your navel, and the third part to the right side of your navel.
3. Raise your forearms to shoulder height, keeping the beaks pointing downward. Slowly open the palms and lower the arms to the sides, then brings your palms to face each other in front of your navel.
4. Place your hands on your navel: men place the right hand on top, women place the left hand on top. Feel the energy you have generated and collect it at the navel. Rest.

TAOIST COSMIC HEALING
Core Practices

⚙ Grasping the Moon: Connecting the Heaven and
Earth Forces

(Pages 104–7)

1. In a standing position, do Bone Marrow Washing and then the Inner Smile meditation.
2. Do the Buddha Palm Opening Movements.
3. Right side Grasping the Moon: With palms facing down, draw the left hand a few inches under the right elbow, leaving the left index finger pointing up toward the right arm's Heart 3. The right index finger points up toward heaven and draws in heavenly force, which cycles through the bones of the right arm, across the shoulders to the left arm, then out the tip of the left index finger into Heart 3 on the right. Keep this energy cycling for 5 seconds.
4. With the arms in the same position, point both index fingers down. The right finger now points toward Large Intestine 11 on the left arm, and the left index finger draws in Earth Chi and Universal Chi. Draw the earth force in through the left index finger up the left arm and across the shoulders down into the right arm and hand. From the right index finger the energy enters Large Intestine 11 on the left and keeps cycling for 5 seconds.

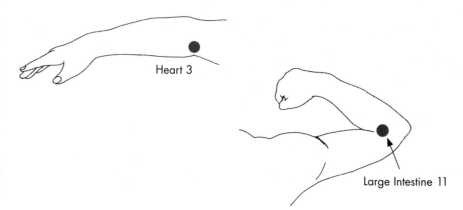

Heart 3

Large Intestine 11

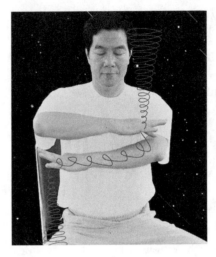

Grasping the Moon

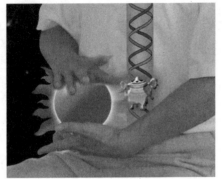

Forming a chi ball

5. Repeat steps 3 and 4 two more times.

6. Right side grasping the chi ball: Hold your left hand in front of the lower tan tien—palm facing up and the pinkie pointing toward the body. Hold your right hand in front of your navel with the palm facing down, as though grasping a small chi ball between the palms. Point your right thumb toward the Laogong point (Pericardium 8) on the left hand, then point it toward your navel.

7. Yin and yang palms: Separate your hands and hold them above your thighs, the left hand still facing up and right hand still facing down. Draw in earth and heaven energies, then turn the left palm over to draw in the earth force through both palms.

8. Repeat steps 1–7 above, switching hands, so that the left arm is over the right. All the right hand instructions now apply to the left hand and vice versa.

9. Finish with the Buddha Palm closing movements.

☯ Opening the Bridge and Regulator Channels
(Pages 108–13)

1. In a standing position, do Bone Marrow Washing and then the Inner Smile meditation.

2. Practice the Buddha Palm opening movements.

3. Place your left palm an inch in front of your throat with the Lung 10 point (in the middle of the mound at the base of the thumb) directly in front of the throat center. Place your right palm an inch behind the left palm, with the Lung 10 points aligned. Feel the chi beaming through your neck and connecting with C7, then with the universe behind your head. Hold for 5–30 seconds, then slowly pull your hands away as if you were pulling silk.

4. Keeping the Lung 10 points aligned, move your hands to 1 inch in front of the mid-eyebrow point. Beam energy through your hands

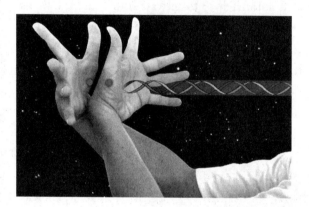

Pulling silk

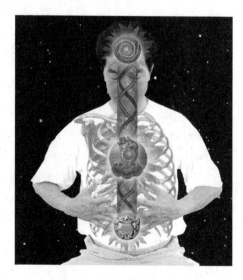

Bridge and Regulator Channels

into the mid-eyebrow point, then through your head to the Jade Pillow and out to the universe behind your head. Hold for 5–30 seconds, then use a small portion of your awareness to pull your hands away like pulling silk. Draw them in again and out 2 more times, then bring them in.

5. Keeping the Lung 10 points aligned, move your hands back down to the throat, then separate the hands to align the Laogong points on the palms (Pericardium 8) with the Stomach 13 points on either side (just below the clavicle, in line with the nipples). The tips of the middle fingers should almost be touching one another. Beam energy from the Laogong points into Stomach 13 to activate your heart and lungs, then beam the energy through your back into the universe. Move your hands down to Stomach 16 (1 inch above the nipples) and beam energy through the heart and middle of the lungs into the universe behind you.

6. Move your hands down to the Liver 14 points (2–3 inches directly below the nipples) and beam healing energy into your liver and gallbladder.

7. Move your hands down to Spleen 16 (just below the ribcage on the mammillary line). Beam healing energy into the stomach, pancreas, spleen, and liver.

8. Move your hands down to Spleen 15 (beside the navel on the mammillary line) and beam healing energy into the small intestine and your lower tan tien.

9. Form a chi ball by lowering your left hand to the level of your lower tan tien and turning your palm upward, pointing your pinkie in toward your body. Face the right palm downward over the left palm, with the Large Intestine 4 point aligned with the navel. Feel the chi ball here and in the tan tien connect to Universal Chi.

10. Repeat steps 3–9 with your right hand at your throat and your left hand behind it. When you form the chi ball in step 9, have your left hand on top and your right hand on the bottom.

11. Finish with the Buddha Palm closing movements.

Opening the Functional Channel
(Pages 114–23)

1. In a standing position, do Bone Marrow Washing and the Inner Smile meditation.
2. Practice the Buddha Palm opening movements.
3. With both palms facing down, align the Pericardium 6 point on your right wrist with the Triple Warmer 5 point on the back of the left wrist, allowing about an inch of space between them. Feel the two points activate each other and hold for 30 seconds. Keeping the wrists crossed, rotate your hands so that the palms are facing up: now the left wrist's Pericardium 6 is aligned with the right wrist's Triple Warmer 5. Hold for 30 seconds, keeping the tan tien and universe spiraling.

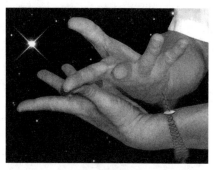

Crossing wrists (TW 5/PC 6)

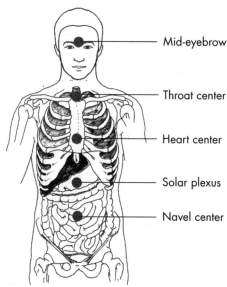

Mid-eyebrow

Throat center

Heart center

Solar plexus

Navel center

Opening the Functional Channel

4. Bring your left hand down to the level of the tan tien, with your palm facing up and the chi knife (index and middle fingers together) pointing toward your body. Make a chi ball by lowering your right hand—palm down—over your left, aligning Large Intestine 4 (the "eye" of the hand) with your navel. Beam energy from Large Intestine 4 into the navel point.

5. Move your right hand up along the Functional Channel, pausing at the solar plexus center to beam energy from Large Intestine 4. While maintaining awareness of the chi ball between your two hands, continue to rise along the channel, pausing to beam energy into the heart center, throat center, and mid-eyebrow point. Then return down the Functional Channel, stopping again at the same energy centers and ending at the navel, holding the chi ball.

6. Double Beam: Turn both palms toward your body, so that the left palm—and its Laogong point—is about an inch away from your navel and the right palm is an inch behind the left, with its Laogong point aligned with the Laogong of the left hand and with the navel. Beam

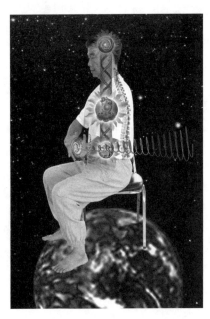

Double beam

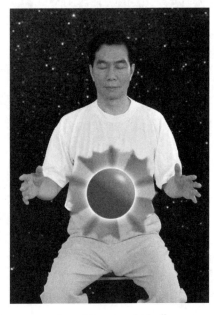

Stretching the chi ball

energy through both Laogong points to the navel and through the body to the Door of Life. Hold for 30 seconds.

7. Draw your left palm up to align its Laogong point with the solar plexus, then bring the right palm up behind the left to align it. Beam energy from both Laogong points into the solar plexus, then through the body to T11.

8. Continue moving your hands upward—left before right—to align with the heart point and the Wing point behind it, then to the throat point and C7, and then to the mid-eyebrow point and the Jade Pillow. Stop at each set of points to beam energy for 30 seconds.

9. Move the left palm then the right palm up to the Crown point. Spiral the palms lightly, letting the chi penetrate deeply into the body, reaching the perineum and opening the Thrusting Channel. (This may take 30–60 seconds.) Then return down the front of the body, with the left hand leading the right, stopping at each energy center to beam energy from the Laogong points.

10. Repeat steps 6–9 two more times. This will activate the Functional, Governor, and Thrusting Channels.

11. Grasping the chi ball: Separate your hands at the level of your navel and hold them in front of you, with palms facing each other. Grasp the chi ball, stretching and squeezing it 3 times, while maintaining awareness of the tan tien and universe spiraling.

12. Repeat steps 3–5 with the left hand over the right, activating all the points on the Functional Channel with the eye of the left hand.

13. Repeat steps 6–10 with your right hand facing your body and your left hand behind it. Then grasp the chi ball and stretch/squeeze it 3 times, remaining aware of the tan tien and universe spiraling.

14. Practice the Buddha Palm closing movements.

Yin and Yang Channels
(Pages 124–29)

1. In a standing position, do Bone Marrow Washing and then the Inner Smile meditation.

2. Practice the Buddha Palm opening movements.

3. Yin channels, left side: In a sitting position, hold your arms in front of you with palms facing down. Turn your right palm over and stroke the air an inch away from the yin channels of your left arm, from palm to armpit. Then pass your right palm an inch away from your body down the left side of your abdomen (along the descending colon) then across the pelvis to the right side.

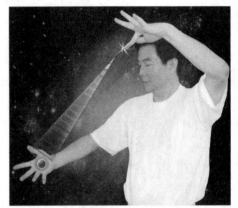

Finger beaming

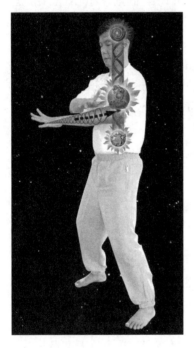

Yang channels

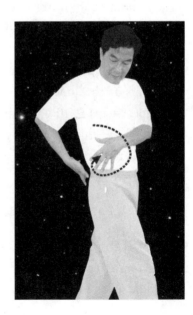

Activating the chi belt

4. Pass your right hand up the right side of your body to the level of your forehead. Turn your left palm face up, then turn your right palm to face the left one. Beam chi from the right palm to the left for 30–60 seconds.

5. Point the ring finger (Triple Warmer channel) of your right hand toward your left palm and make small circles with it, beaming chi to the left hand for 30–60 seconds. Return the ring finger to a neutral position. Now point the left ring finger up toward the right palm and project chi for 30–60 seconds. Return the left ring finger to a neutral position. Point both ring fingers toward the opposite palm and project chi from both fingers for 30–60 seconds, noticing that the energy may meet in the middle. Return fingers to neutral.

6. Yang channels, left side: Turn your left palm down and hold your right palm 1 inch away from the back of your left hand. Pass your right palm over the outside of the left arm from the hand to the shoulder. Next pass your right palm across your upper chest and right breast. Scoop the right palm under your right armpit, then bring the right palm forward, palm down. Press forward with your left palm at the same time, then relax and channel the earth force.

7. Repeat steps 3–6 on the right side of your body with the hands reversed.

8. Repeat steps 3–7 four more times, using a different pair of fingers each time to beam chi. First use your index fingers (Large Intestine channel), then your thumbs (Lung channel), then your pinkies (Heart channel), and finally your middle fingers (Pericardium channel).

9. Belt Channel: Step forward with your right foot as you place your right palm over your navel and your left palm over the Door of Life. Feel the chi beam penetrate from palm to palm. Turn your hips to the right and shift weight to your right leg. At the same time, move your right palm to the Door of Life and your left palm to your right hip in a sweeping manner.

10. Repeat step 9 two more times, then reverse all hand and foot directions and repeat 3 more times with your left foot forward.

11. Practice the Buddha Palm closing movements.

CHI NEI TSANG

🌀 Healing Hands Meditation

(Pages 69–77)

🌸 Part 1: Meditating to Expand the Aura

1. Practice the Inner Smile meditation, then bring energy to your navel center. Practice the Fusion meditations, forming four pakuas and transforming negative emotions into positive healing forces. Then form a pearl.

2. Circulate the pearl in your Microcosmic Orbit faster and faster until it expands outward from your body, filling your aura with a warm sensation. Absorb violet and red lights from the North Star and the Big Dipper above you; absorb golden light from the cosmic particle energy; absorb blue light from the earth into your navel.

3. When your aura has expanded, maintain a distance of at least 2 feet from other people.

🌸 Part 2: Channeling Force through the Palms

4. Hold both hands in front of your eyes and use the corners of both eyes to gaze at the palms' centers. Use your mind and eyes to absorb Cosmic Chi into your right palm, then send the chi from your right palm and fingers into your left palm and fingers. Repeat 9 times.

5. Hold your hands facing each other but not touching, and feel the energy travel between them. Gradually spread your hands apart while maintaining the chi connection between them. Pull them together and apart 9–18 times.

🌸 Parts 3 and 4: Growing the Auras of Your Fingers

6. With both palms facing your eyes, gaze from the corners of the right eye at the right hand's fingers. Focus on the tip of the index finger and its aura. Using the energy of your eyes, expand the aura of this fingertip, making the energy cool and pleasant. Then grow the auras of your other fingers in turn: middle finger, thumb, ring finger, and pinkie.

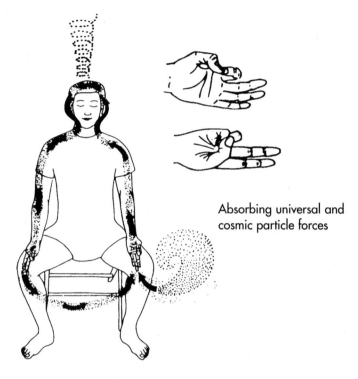

Absorbing universal and
cosmic particle forces

7. Inhale energy into your left hand and fingers, and gaze at the tip of
your thumb. Grow the thumb's aura, then turn your gaze to each of
the other fingers, growing the auras of the index finger, middle finger,
ring finger, and pinkie finger.

8. Place your palms up on your knees. On your left hand, form a circle
with your thumb and index finger, keeping the other fingers straight.
On your right hand, form a circle with your thumb and the ring and
pinkie fingers, keeping the index and middle fingers straight.

9. Keeping your fingers in these circles, use your mind and eyes to absorb
cosmic particle force through the fingers of the left hand. Send it up
the outside of the left arm and shoulder to the back of the left ear and
across the crown. Blend this energy with the universal force entering
through the crown, then send this combined energy down to the right
ear, right shoulder, the outside of the right arm and hand, and then
to the index and middle fingers. Send this energy out through these
fingers and receive it again through the extended fingers of the left
hand. Repeat for 18 or 36 cycles.

⚙ Fanning Hot Sick Energy
(Pages 107–9)

1. In a sitting position, raise your left hand to the level of your heart (about 1.5 inches from the top of the sternum), with the palm facing downward. Place your right palm an inch or so above your left hand, aligning the Laogong points (Pericardium 8). Practice the heart's sound (haw-w-w-w-w-w) and feel the heat from the heart start to burn, drawing in any negative feelings.

2. Exhale this energy using the heart's sound as you lower both hands, feeling the negative energies burn out. Exhale the energy down to the perineum, the backs of the feet, and the soles, allowing Mother Earth to absorb it.

3. Rest for a while with your palms on your knees, then repeat the above steps 18–36 times, for a total of 5–10 minutes. You may begin to feel empty, but good. Allow your body to fill with the golden light of heavenly energy coming down through your crown and the blue light of Mother Earth energy coming up through the soles of your feet.

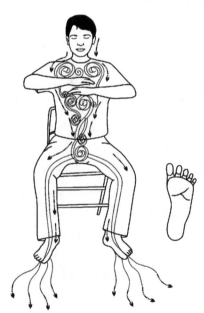

Fanning sick energy from the heart to the soles of the feet

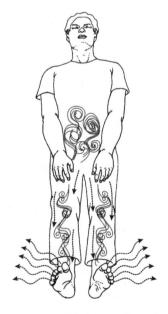

Venting sick energy from the fingers and toes

⚙ Venting Hot Sick Energy

(Pages 109–15)

1. Sit with your hands on your knees, fingers slightly spread and pointing toward your toes. Have your feet parallel to each other with the toes pointing upward. Exhale the triple warmer's sound (hee-e-e-e-e) down to the navel, perineum, and toes.

2. Notice a steaming, dark, cloudy, or chilly sick energy emerging from your fingers and toes. Picture the energy becoming brighter. Focus your awareness on your liver and see it become a bright green, then see your spleen and pancreas begin to glow with a bright yellow color. See the lungs glow with a bright white light and the heart open with bright red light. Focus on your kidneys and watch them glow with a bright blue light.

3. Repeat steps 1 and 2 nine times.

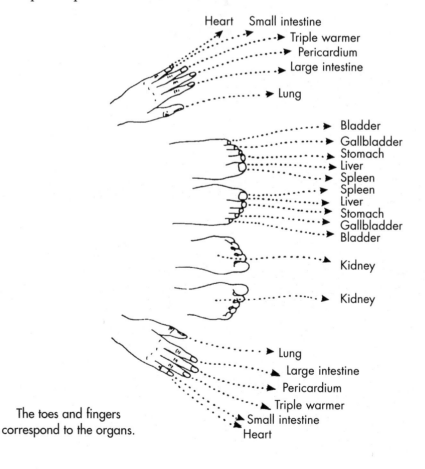

The toes and fingers correspond to the organs.

CHI NEI TSANG

◔ Opening the Wind Gates

(Pages 146–59)

Use the table of Wind Gate pulse counts below to determine how many pulse-beats to count as you hold each point.

1. Groin: Press the edge of each palm into the femoral artery pulse at the crease of each leg. Hold for 36 or 72 counts of the pulse.

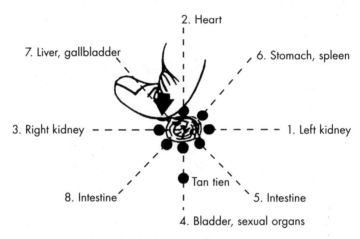

Wind gate points on the sides of the navel

PULSE COUNTS FOR OPENING THE WIND GATES

Day	Tan tien point below navel	point 1	point 2	point 3	point 4	point 5	point 6	point 7	point 8
Monday	15	8	17	19	21	10	12	6	15
Tuesday	8	17	19	21	10	12	6	15	8
Wednesday	17	19	21	10	12	6	15	8	17
Thursday	19	21	10	12	6	15	8	17	19
Friday	21	10	12	6	15	8	17	19	21
Saturday	10	12	6	15	8	17	19	21	10
Sunday	6	15	8	17	19	21	10	12	6

2. Tan Tien: Locate the tan tien pressure point in a depression about 1.5 inches below the navel. Press in with your thumb or elbow—angling toward the left side of the tan tien—until you feel the aortic pulse. Hold for the number of pulse-beats indicated in the table for this day.
3. Navel Wind Gate points: Use your thumb to press with moderate pressure into each wind gate point until you feel the pulse. Hold for the number of pulse beats indicated in the chart, then release. Work on point 1 (left kidney) first, then point 2 (heart) and the other points in order: 3 (right kidney), 4 (bladder and genitals), 5 (intestines), 6 (spleen and stomach), 7 (liver), 8 (intestines).
4. Relax and pat lightly around the navel to complete the session.

🌀 Chasing the Winds
(Pages 157–48)

1. Use the one-finger technique to spiral around the navel.
2. Baking hot wind: Place both hands over the small intestine and chant the heart's sound with your student (haw-w-w-w-w-w). Feel heat and pressure in the small intestine, then move your left hand to the student's lower back—opposite your right hand. Chant the heart's sound again to move or cook the wind.
3. Baking cold wind: Place your right hand on the cold wind and your left hand on the small intestine. Chant the kidneys' sound (Choo-oo-oo-oo) with your student to build the wind into a cold ball in the small intestine. Move one hand to your student's lower back, and chant the heart's sound together to bake the wind thoroughly. Tap around the navel with your fingertips or scratch the affected area lightly to help purge these winds.
4. Burning sick wind: Use the scooping technique* to scoop sick energy into the lower tan tien. Notice a cold or chilly energy forming there. Use your index and middle fingers to press on this area while your student concentrates on this point. Spiral with your fingers to generate a "sunshine" heat in this spot that gradually displaces the cold, sick wind.

---

*Details on the scooping technique can be found in *Chi Nei Tsang,* page 165.

CHI NEI TSANG

🌀 Navel Diagnosis and Release

(Pages 117–22)

1. Make the navel round, then release it and see where it pulls. This indicates the tight area that needs to be loosened.
2. Press the area around the navel with your thumb or elbow and loosen it slowly. Repeat up to 3 times.
3. Shape and round the navel into a perfect circle, then hold it like this for a few moments to release tensions.

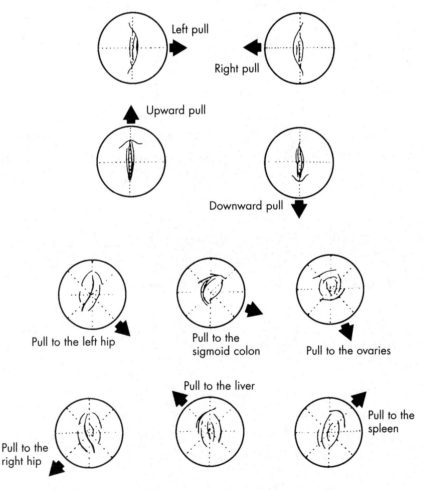

Chi Nei Tsang navel examination

Upward pull: May cause problems with: intestines, menstruation, constipation, prostate, heartburn, breathing, insomnia, and/or cough.

Pull to the upper right: May affect the liver, gallbladder, lower left hip, left leg, and/or the intestines.

Pull to the upper left: May affect the lower right hip and right leg, and/or the stomach and spleen, causing digestive problems.

Pull to the right: May affect the left side, kidneys, or intestines.

Leftward pull: May affect the right side, the kidneys, and/or the intestines.

Right hip pull: Causes tension on the upper left side of navel. Affects the pancreas, stomach, spleen, and left kidney. May also give rise to pain in the lumbar plexus or the right leg.

Left hip pull: Creates tension and pain on the upper right side of the navel. May cause problems with the gallbladder, duodenum, or right kidney; can also create pain in the lumbar plexus or left leg.

Downward pull: May cause intestinal pain, mental health issues, bad dreams, menstrual problems, or symptoms of the prostate or bladder.

Eight directions of possible pulls on the navel

CHI NEI TSANG
Detoxifying the Skin and the Large and Small Intestines

❂ Detoxifying the Skin
(Pages 161–68)

1. Spiraling: Using both thumbs or forefingers together, gently massage a point at the edge of the navel in small, tight, clockwise circular motions, loosening the skin. Work outward in a spiral from the navel to the edges of the abdomen, massaging point by point.
2. Scooping: With your fingers together, press inwardly and scoop in, or press downward and scoop out.
3. Rocking: Spread your fingers to cover the ascending and descending colon, or bring them together to cover the small intestine. Use all your fingers to hold the abdominal muscles while rocking your hands back and forth.
4. Shaking: Press on a knot or problem area with your index or middle finger. Vibrate your finger rapidly up and down or from side to side.
5. Patting: Pat around the navel and entire abdominal area with your fingers and a soft open palm.

❂ Detoxifying the Large Intestine
(Pages 169–85)

1. Figure-Five technique: Stand or sit at your student's right side and work on the left side. Using both palms, stroke upward along the midline toward the sternum, then forcefully brush the left ribcage toward the sternum. Place your right thumb below the nipple between the eighth and ninth ribs and stroke downward to a point level with the point midway between the sternum and the navel. Make a wide half circle under the left ribcage, following the descending colon and ending at the sigmoid colon.

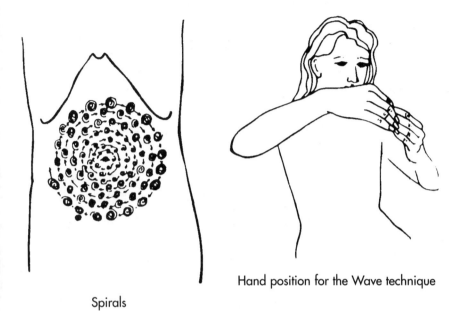

Spirals

Hand position for the Wave technique

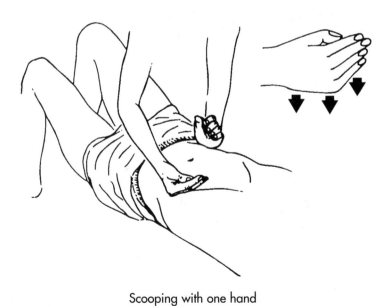

Scooping with one hand

2. Wave technique: Cup your hands with the fingertips overlapping, then press into the abdomen. With the edge of your left palm, press inward and slide upward along the ascending colon. Rock along the edges of your hands to cross the transverse colon, then press the edge of your right hand in and slide downward along the descending colon. Repeat several times.

3. Releasing the sigmoid colon: Sitting at your student's left side, have her raise her left knee. Place the edge of your right hand against her left hip bone and the fingertips of your left hand on top of the pubic bone. Press with the edge of your right hand underneath (not on top of) the sigmoid colon. Roll out from under it with the back of your hand moving toward the rib cage. Repeat this motion several times, then do the Wave technique 3–6 times.

4. Releasing the cecum: Use one finger to press around the right hip and feel for a bulge—about an inch long—under the ileocecal valve. Press your thumbs firmly into this point and use a consistent pressure to inch up toward the ileocecal valve. Repeat 2 or 3 times.

5. Opening a stuck ileocecal valve: Place the edge of your right hand along the right hip bone and your left hand on the back behind the kidneys. Slowly apply downward pressure with the edge of your right hand, then roll your palm diagonally up toward the ribcage. Do not repeat more than once.

6. Closing an open ileocecal valve: Do a counterclockwise Wave technique by moving upward along the descending colon. Rock counterclockwise along the transverse colon, then slide your hands downward along the ascending colon.

Detoxifying the Small Intestine
(Pages 185–92)

If the student's abdomen is very tight and sensitive, you will have to loosen it gently before undertaking deeper work. Allow your fingers to just skim over the abdomen, or lay your palm on the skin and gently spiral it.

1. Begin with the Wave technique, feeling for knots and areas of tension. Then use the basic spiraling technique to massage the small intestine, trying to follow the many curves in this organ. Gently vibrate your finger into any tight areas, working in short bursts with both clockwise and counterclockwise spirals. Always pull your fingers and any released energy toward the cecum, where the contents of the small intestine flow into the large intestine.

2. Work until you have massaged the whole small intestine, then cover it with your hands and have the student breathe into your hands. Practice the Inner Smile meditation with your student.

⟳ Releasing Knots, Tangles, and Nerves
(Pages 193–97)

Knots are muscle knots that can build pressure against the nerves and lymph nodes. Tangles are deeper than knots and consist of nerves and arteries that are twisted together, often with lymph nodes and fatty tissue inside them. Knots and tangles can take many sessions to resolve.

1. Knots: Press down gently on the knot and spiral. You may wish to begin with your palm or palm-heel, then progress to three fingers, two fingers, one finger. If the abdomen is very tight and knotted, work on a looser area first, gradually extending the relaxed area until you have worked all the way around the knot. Then work on the knot directly. Teach your student how to continue this work at home.

2. Tangles: Loosen the whole abdomen, practice skin detoxification techniques, and relax any knots. Then work at the edges of the tangle until it begins to unravel. Slowly work toward the center.

3. Untangling nerves: Where there is numbness from a tangle of nerves, first work the tangle upward away from the navel. If this does not change the condition, work downward toward the navel.

4. End with the patting technique.

CHI NEI TSANG
Detoxifying the Organs

Releasing the Diaphragm
(Pages 199–207)

1. Begin by massaging around the navel, then releasing and stimulating the large intestine as shown on pages 160–62 of this book.
2. Place one hand on the left side of the ribcage. While your student inhales, slide your other hand beneath the left ribs to lift them. While

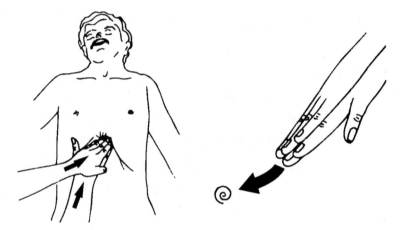

Releasing the diaphragm using both hands

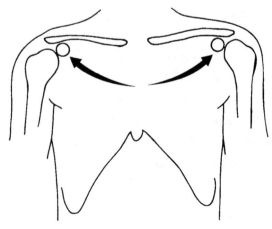

Lung 1 points

the student exhales, press down with your hand on top of the rib cage. Repeat on the right side.

3. Press your fingers down along the edges of the rib cage, beginning at the lower left and ending at the lower right.

4. Spiral your thumbs along the edge of the bottom rib, beginning at the lower right edge and working up toward the sternum. At the bottom of the sternum use two or three fingers to spiral, then one hand on top of the other to release the diaphragm here. Spiral with your thumbs again as you work down the edge of the lowest rib on the left side.

✷ Detoxifying the Lungs

(Pages 225–28)

Be sure to release any congestion in the splenic band under the left rib cage before detoxifying the lungs. Use the Figure-Five technique outlined on page 160.

1. Press your fingertips firmly into the left Lung 1 point. Have the student breathe the lungs' sound (sss-s-s-s-s-s) into your finger a few times, until you feel a pulsing at the point.

2. With one hand on the left upper rib cage (above the breast) and the other hand below the breast, have your student inhale using deep abdominal breathing. When the lungs are full, rock the rib cage, then push it toward the right side as the student exhales. Let the student take another complete breath as you press gently but firmly on the rib cage during exhalation, rocking it if you like.

3. Repeat the previous step 3–5 times.

4. Repeat the hand position from step 2, but this time have the student inhale then exhale completely, and rock the ribcage after the exhalation. Hold your pressure on the rib cage as the student inhales the next breath, rocking if you like, and let the student exhale. Repeat 3–5 times. On the last inhalation reduce the pressure of your hands but stay in contact with the student's chest. Allow the lungs to overfill with air.

5. Repeat steps 1–4 on the right side.

☯ Detoxifying the Spleen
(Pages 228–30)

1. First do the Figure-Five technique to release any congestion at the splenic bend.
2. Use your thumbs or fingers to spiral in the spleen area under the left rib cage. Add weight by pressing down on your fingers with your other hand. You should not encounter any hardness because the spleen is soft tissue, but take the time to work on it at length.
3. Have your student push away your fingers with his or her Spleen Chi.
4. Use the Baking technique with one hand on top of the spleen and the other beneath it (on the back).

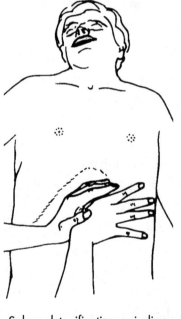

Spleen detoxification: spiraling with the thumbs

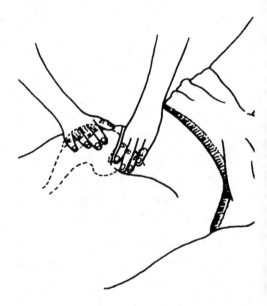

Pumping the spleen, stomach, and pancreas

❂ Detoxifying the Pancreas
(Pages 230–33)

1. Stand or kneel at the student's right side and place the "knife edge" of your hand on the head of the pancreas at the midline, pressing as deeply into it as your student can tolerate.
2. Have your student make the spleen's sound (who-o-o-o-o-o) as you apply a rolling pressure along the edge of your hand, pumping toward the midline so that stones or crystals do not enter the spleen.
3. Pumping technique: Place one hand on top of the lower part of the left rib cage, pressing down to help exhalation. With your other hand, massage under the ribs as your student exhales. Massage your way under the ribs, pumping toward the body's midline and scooping toward the navel.

❂ Detoxifying the Liver
(Pages 233–43)

1. First clear the large intestine and work on the rib cage, diaphragm, spleen, and pancreas.
2. Bake the liver by holding your left hand on the student's back, opposite the lower right rib cage, and your right hand on the right side of the abdomen over the liver. Bake the liver between your hands.

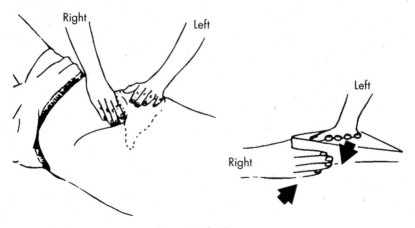

Pumping the liver

3. Make small, circular motions with your fingertips on the liver, searching for hardened spots and spending additional time on these. Have your student make the liver's sound (sh-h-h-h-h-h-h) throughout this exercise, and breathe directly into any tension.

4. For the lower part of the liver, place your thumbs beneath the lower right side of the ribcage, letting your fingers rest gently on the ribs. Press in and rock upward with both thumbs under the right rib cage, then scoop the thumbs in and down, creating a pumping action and releasing the lower edge of the liver. Move along the lower border of the rib cage, making small circles as you work up toward the common bile duct. Loosen any knots or tightness.

5. For the middle lobe of the liver, use the same thumb technique, changing the angle of the thumbs as needed to contact more of the liver tissue.

6. To work on the upper part of the liver, place your hands to the right of the xiphoid process, one on top of the other. Use your fingertips to work underneath the ribs, sweeping toward the gallbladder. This part of the liver lies just below the heart; have your student make the heart's sound (haw-w-w-w-w-w) as you work on this area, returning to the liver's sound as you work on other parts of the liver.

7. When finished, ask you student to push your fingers away using his or her liver and chi.

8. Pump the liver by placing your right palm just below right rib cage, with your fingers pointing into the left rib cage. Place your left hand on top of the right ribs and pump it several times toward the navel or the left hip. Coordinate with your student's exhalations and rock your body to create the movement.

☋ Detoxifying the Kidneys
(Pages 242–49)

1. Have your student lie on her back and rotate her lower body toward the left, so that the right leg is on top of the left leg, and the right hip is pointing straight up. Bend the right knee.
2. Use all your fingers to look for the right kidney—press your fingers deep toward the spine about 1 inch from the navel, extending upward to the ribcage. Massage the kidney gently with spiraling finger techniques. Have the student make the kidneys' sound with each exhalation. Work for 1–2 minutes, even less if the massage is painful.
3. Have the student push your fingers out of the kidney with her chi.
4. Blow warm air into the right kidney from a distance of 2–3 inches, then bake the kidney between your hands.
5. Repeat steps 1–4 on the other side to work on the left kidney.
6. Detoxify the bladder area by moving your fingers or thumbs in small circles until the area feels free of congestion and pain.

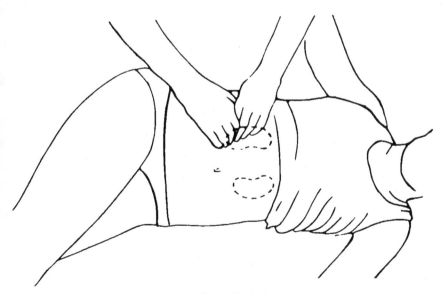

Detoxifying the kidneys

🌀 Detoxifying the Heart and Heart Protector (Pericardium)

(Pages 259–60)

1. Massage the heart area with one hand while pressing Heart 7 on the wrist with the other hand. Have your student exhale the heart's sound.
2. Have your student continue making the heart's sound as you massage the heart protector area with one hand and the Pericardium 6 point with your other hand.

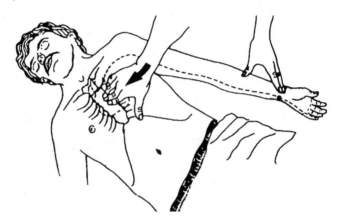

Detoxifying the heart

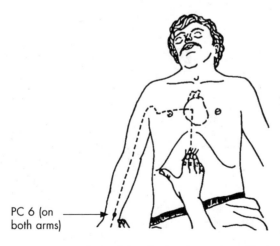

PC 6 (on both arms)

Detoxifying the heart protector (Pericardium)

CHI NEI TSANG

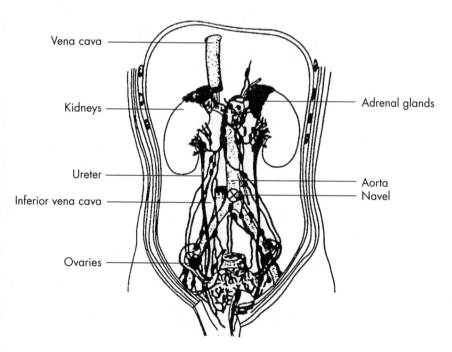

Releasing Toxins from the Lymph System
(Pages 253–67)

1. Massage the navel, first clockwise and then counterclockwise, then do the Wave technique until you can reach deep into the abdomen. Feel for lymph nodes along the midline (they are smaller than knots or tangles) and massage them lightly with your fingertips. Continue searching the abdomen for additional nodes, especially around the aorta and vena cava. Massage any palpable nodes.

2. Place your hands flat on your student's navel and ask him to breathe against them while you press down. When the student exhales, press down a little more to activate the lymph flow into the thoracic duct.

3. Place your thumbs underneath the lower ribs at the level of the liver and push them gently upward and toward the midline, stroking the ribs as you go. Continue to the bottom of the sternum.

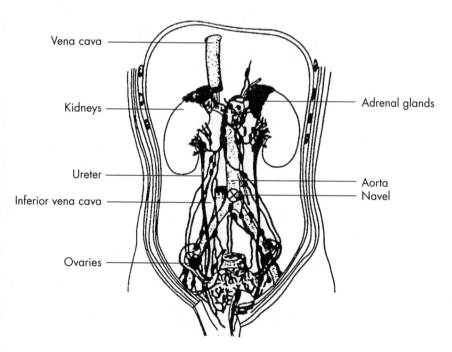

Lymphatic pathways in the kidneys, aorta, and lower abdomen

4. Place your fingertips between the ribs on the left side of the ribcage at the sternum. Beginning with the lower ribs, massage in downward circles, pushing the lymph into the body toward the thoracic duct. Work your way up the rib cage to the clavicle, then repeat on the right side.

5. Drain the areas above the collarbone into the vena cava by placing your middle and index fingers on the upper border of the collarbone and massaging in downward circles.

6. Standing at your student's head, use your fingertips to massage below the ear, down the jawline, and down the side of the neck. Use the same downward circular motion to drain the fluid into the spaces above the collarbones. You can work on one or both sides at a time,

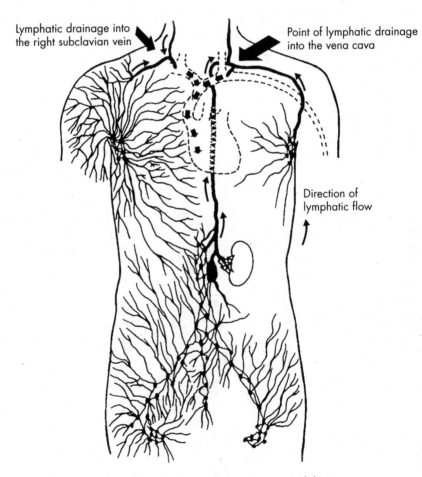

Lymphatic drainage into the right subclavian vein

Point of lymphatic drainage into the vena cava

Direction of lymphatic flow

Lymphatic drainage into the right subclavian vein and the vena cava but do not massage nodes in this area that are enlarged or painful.

7. With flat hands, press the lymph nodes in each armpit downward into the body. Again, do not massage any lymph nodes that are enlarged or painful.

8. With flattened hands or your fingers, press the groin nodes toward the lower abdomen collection point near the second lumbar vertebra.

9. End by placing the student's hands over his navel and inviting him to rest. Thank the lymph nodes for allowing you to work on them.

Balancing the Pulses
(Pages 274–85)

Work on the pulses on the left side of the body first, then those on the right side. Do not perform these massages on anyone with detached retinas, diabetes, heart problems, thromboses, or varicose veins. Do not perform on pregnant women.

1. Standing at the student's left side, hold the aorta with your left hand while placing one or two fingers of your right hand on the left carotid. Feel the pulses, and gently hold them until they are synchronized.

2. Maintain your hold on the aorta while you locate the pulse in the left armpit with the fingers of your right hand. Hold the two pulses until they are balanced.

3. Place the fingers of your right hand on the pulse in the crease of the left elbow. Balance it with the aortic pulse, then balance the radial pulse in the left wrist with the aortic pulse.

4. Now hold the aortic pulse with your right hand and use your left hand to find the pulse at the left femoral artery, just below the crease of the thigh and pelvis. Hold and balance these two major arteries.

5. Keeping your right hand on the aortic pulse, move your left hand underneath the left knee. Feel for the popliteal pulse just below the crease of the knee. Allow this pulse to synchronize to the aortic pulse.

6. Move your left hand to the inside ankle bone and locate the pulse just below the ankle joint. Hold this pulse until it adjusts to the aortic pulse.

7. Repeat steps 1–6 on the right side of the body.

CHI NEI TSANG
Working on the Sexual Organs

⟳ Uterus and Ovaries

(Pages 310–17)

1. Uterus massage: Place your thumbs together on one side of the uterus and all of your fingers on the other side, keeping your hands aligned. Apply a deep, probing, kneading motion to massage any tangles or twists, then hold the uterus with both hands for a few moments.

2. Use techniques for removing winds to clear any heat that may be causing tangles in the uterus and fallopian tubes, then use detoxification techniques to clear any congestion in this area. Cup your hands between the ovaries, push in gently, and massage the area above the cervix. Massage the fallopian tubes with gentle, circular motions.

3. Ovary massage: Standing at your student's right side, massage the ovaries by rocking between the heel and fingers of your hand. The heel of your hands massages the right ovary and your fingers massage the left ovary. Continue for 5 minutes or longer, pushing and pumping with a soft rock and roll motion. Repeat on the left side.

4. Teach your student how to work on herself at home to maintain the benefits of this massage.

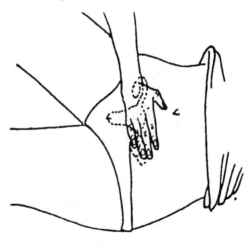

Ovarian Massage

Prostate

(Pages 317–18)

1. First work on the liver. Check for knots and tangles in the lower abdomen and along the creases of the legs. Massage gently.

2. Teach student to do testicle and duct massage, as described on pages 88–90. Pull the urethra out from the perineum and squeeze it to loosen plaque formations.

3. Work just above the pubic bone, massaging in circles with two fingers. At the depression directly above the bladder and prostate, work a little longer.

4. Find the hole where the testicles ascend and descend. Insert a finger into this hole to loosen any knots or tangles.

5. Massage the prostate, which is right above the perineum, just under the skin between the anus and the testicles.

6. Bake and massage the kidneys and adrenal glands.

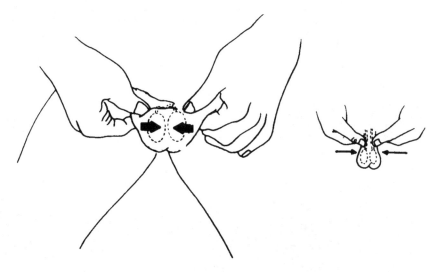

Teach your student to massage and elongate the ducts.

CHI NEI TSANG
Treating Common Ailments

✪ Tension Headaches

(Pages 301–5)

1. Work on the navel then use both thumbs to massage down the sides of the cervical and brachial vertebrae, then work on the brachial plexus, releasing knots and tangles.
2. With student lying face down, place the back of his right hand on the spine, and hold it there gently. Use your thumb to massage the scapula muscle underneath the right shoulder blade.
3. Grasp the trapezius muscle between your thumb and fingers, and massage it toward the shoulder, then use two thumbs to massage straight down the right side of the spine.
4. Repeat steps 2 and 3 on the left side of the spine.
5. To relieve and acute tension headache, detoxify the skin and release the large intestine. Then detoxify the liver, gallbladder, and kidneys. Work on the adrenal glands.

✪ Lower Back Pain

(Pages 288–92)

🌸 Releasing the Sciatic Nerve

1. With student on her back, rotate the hips in their sockets, then place the student on her left side. Use your thumb or elbow to massage piriformis muscle in the hip hole.
2. Massage down the midline of the back of the thigh, then use your thumbs to massage on both sides of the knee. Use your fingers to move the popliteal tendons apart.
3. Massage under the inner ankle bone near Kidney 3, then raise the lower leg and tap the heel with your fist.
4. Repeat steps 1–3 on the other leg.

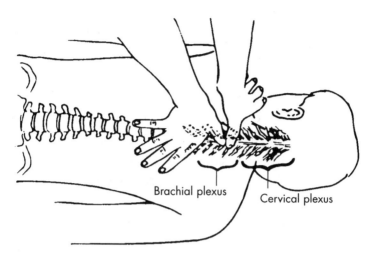

Massage the brachial and cervical
plexi to treat headaches.

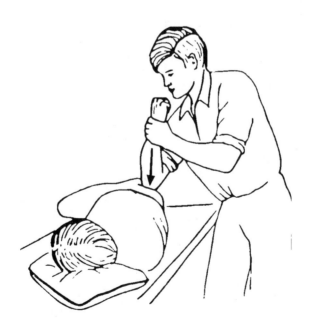

For releasing sciatic nerve pain, use your
elbow to massage the piriformis muscle.

❀ Releasing the Psoas Muscle

1. Begin with skin detoxification techniques to detoxify the large and small intestines, then loosen any knots or tangles in the lower abdomen and pelvic area.

2. Locate the psoas muscle by having your student raise her knee toward the chest, then rotate it back and forth. While she does this, press your fingers into the area of the psoas muscle until you feel it moving beneath your fingers. Then press all of your fingers down into the muscle, locking onto it as your student lowers her foot to the floor, keeping the knee slightly bent.

3. Press down and hold your fingers still as you shake your body vigorously to the left and right, generating a massage movement in your fingers.

4. Repeat steps 2 and 3 on the other side.

5. Massage the psoas tendons by kneeling beside your student with her lower leg cradled between your arm and neck. Reach into the lower psoas area and find the tendon, which attaches the bottom of the psoas to the top of the femur. Gently move your shoulder toward your student's head to raise the leg a bit, thereby stretching the tendon. Massage and gently pull on the tendon as it stretches, then let it relax. Repeat this massage several times on both sides.

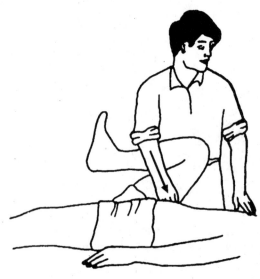

Go in deeply to locate the psoas muscle.

CHI NEI TSANG
Tree Chi Kung

⟳ Using the Palms to Absorb Yin Energy
and Help Balance Yang Energy
(Pages 87–92)

1. Stand or sit 1–2 feet in front of a tree and let your energy field open like a flower.
2. Extend your arms facing your palms toward the tree offering welcome, and breathe in any energy the tree offers you in return. Focus your eyes on the tip of your nose and on your palms at the tree. Use

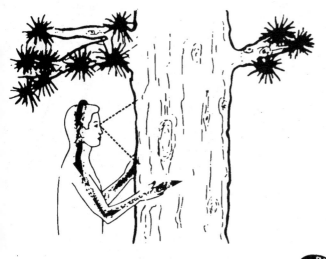

Tree Chi Kung

3. Around the ear

4. Down the inner arm

2. Up the inner arm

5. Back to the tree

1. From the tree

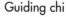

Guiding chi

your left palm, your mind, and the upper part of your eyes to absorb tree chi.

3. Parallel tracking: Control your own energy, and watch the tree while it controls its own energy and watches you.

4. Draw and hold close: Allow the energy field between you and the tree to intensify and thicken, holding you closely together. Hold the tree in a mutual embrace of deep intimacy.

5. Guide the chi: Feel the tree's cool, healing energy as it enters your body. Guide it with the upper part of your eyes up the inside of your left arm to the shoulder, neck, left ear, and crown, then down the right side of the ear, neck, shoulder, right arm, and the right palm. Combine this energy with cosmic particle (human plane) energy and project it out into the tree trunk. Women should repeat this yin energy cycle 24 times, men 36 times.

6. Exchange at a deeper level: Place part of your body in contact with part of the tree's body, and circulate energy back and forth between you, guiding it with your eyes as before.

7. Draw back: Gradually withdraw your attention from contact with the tree and return it to yourself. "Push back" at any shared energy trying to enter your body, allowing your human energy to return to you but not the tree's energy.

8. Allow the tree energy to flow back into the tree as you keep your own energy within your body.

9. Close: Perform a closing gesture like a hand clap, head nod, "Amen," or any other connection-breaking action. End with a little wave or a quick kiss on the trunk.

Absorb Tree Chi through the Yin Side
(Pages 93–95)

1. Stand or sit 1–2 feet in front of a tree with your palms facing it. Absorb the chi of the tree through your palms and guide it up the yin sides of both arms to the shoulders, neck, ears, and crown.

2. From the crown move the energy down the Functional Channel to

the mid-eyebrow, throat, heart, solar plexus, navel, and the lower
tan tien/cauldron, then down to the perineum, soles of the feet, and
approximately 10 feet into the ground.

3. Bring the energy up into the roots of the tree and then into the tree
trunk. Feel your energy flow through the tree and emerge from the
trunk into your palms. Repeat this cycle 24 or 36 times.

4. Send energy from your right palm through the tree's trunk to the left
palm, then reverse. Men should repeat this cycle 36 times, women 24.

5. Send your energy into the upper part of the trunk, then kneel down
to practice with the lower trunk, then practice with the roots of the
tree. Each time exhange force with the tree.

6. End the exercise by drawing back your energy and closing, as in steps
7–9 above.

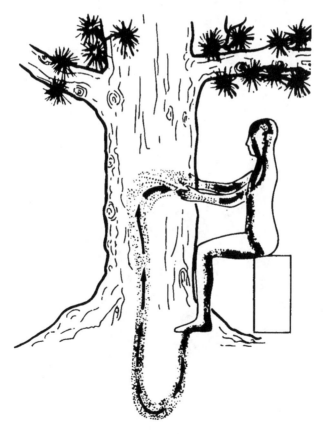

Circulating tree chi through the soles, trunk, and palms.

COSMIC FUSION

🌀 Forming the Pakuas

(Pages 46–67)

Chant each trigram's name and lines in long deep sounds. Always begin with the line closest to the center and move outward.

Each time you chant a yin line, begin with your mind expanded and your hands and palms expanded to touch the cosmos. As you chant *yin yin yin* feel your palms and Cosmic Chi from the universe being drawn down the front of your body to the navel.

Each time you chant a yang line, be aware of the tan tien, throat, and crown. Hold your palms close to the navel and chant the long *yang yang yang* sound as you move your hands out to the right and left sides. Feel them reach out to touch the Cosmic Chi.

1. Chant *Kan* (water) several times as you picture the symbol and touch your lower abdomen.

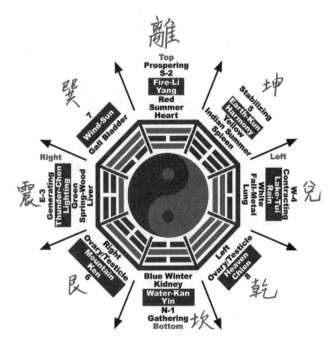

Later Heaven yang pakua

2. Chant the trigram lines—*yin, yang, yin*—with the hand motions as described above.

3. With eyes looking at your lower abdomen, repeat the word *Kan* several times and picture the trigram on your abdomen. Picture the gathering power of yin, water, the kidneys, ears, and sexual organs. Project the trigram into the universe, then feel the Kan symbol in the universe reinforcing the Kan in the abdomen.

4. Chant *Li* (fire) as you picture the symbol and touch your upper abdomen. Feel your energy rise and your eyes look upward as you chant. Next chant the trigram lines—*yang, yin, yang*—expanding and contracting as described above. Repeat the word *Li* as you imprint the Li symbol on your abdomen. Be aware of your heart, tongue, and the prospering power of fire. Project the Li symbol out into the universe, then feel it reinforcing the Li in your abdomen.

5. Chant *Chen* (thunder and lightning) as you picture the symbol on the right side of your abdomen. Let your eyes look to the right. Chant the lines—*yang, yin, yin*—as you expand and contract and picture the liver, the eyes, the wood element, and thunder and lightning power. Repeat the word *Chen* and imprint the trigram on your abdomen, then project it out into the universe.

6. Chant *Tui* (lake) as you picture the symbol on the left side of your abdomen. Eyes look to the left. Chant the lines—*yang, yang, yin*—as you bring your awareness to your lungs and nose, the metal element, and contracting power. Chant *Tui* again and imprint the symbol on your abdomen, then project it out into the universe.

7. Look at each trigram again and repeat its lines, then chant *Kan, Li, Chen, Tui* as you move your eyes down, up, right, and left. Repeat several times. Spiral your fingers around your navel and chant *Tai Chi, Tai Chi, Tai Chi* until you feel the symbol spiraling in the middle of the pakua, like a fire burning inside of you.

8. Chant *Kun* (earth) repeatedly, picturing the symbol on your forehead. Connect with the stomach, spleen, mouth, pancreas, and the stabilizing power of harmony. Chant the lines—*yin, yin, yin*—as you contract your hands. Picture the Kun in front of you and expand it

out to connect with the stabilizing power in the cosmos. Let the cosmic energy return to you, sticking to your forehead, then bring the trigram down to the upper left corner of your abdomen.

9. Chant *Ken* (mountain) repeatedly, picturing the symbol on your forehead. Connect with the bladder, the right sexual organs, and the back of the skull. Chant the lines—*yin, yin, yang*—as you contract and expand your hands. Picture the Ken and expand it out to connect with the stabilizing power of mountain in the cosmos. Let the cosmic energy return to you, sticking to your forehead, then bring the trigram down to the lower right corner of your abdomen.

10. Chant *Sun* (wind) repeatedly, drawing the symbol on the upper right corner of your abdomen. Connect with the the gallbladder and the base of your skull. Chant the lines—*yin, yang, yang*—as you contract and expand your hands. Project the Sun out into the cosmos to connect with the cosmic power of wind. Let the cosmic energy return to you, sticking to your abdomen, then place the trigram in the upper right corner of your abdomen.

11. Chant *Chien* (heaven) repeatedly, marking the symbol on your abdomen. Connect with the large intestine, the forehead bone, and the left sexual organs. Chant the lines—*yang, yang, yang*—as you expand your hands. Picture the Chien in front of you and expand it very far away to connect with the power of heaven. Let the cosmic energy return to you and stick to your abdomen, then bring the trigram down to the lower left corner of your abdomen.

12. Repeat step 7 with all eight trigrams, chanting *Kan, Li, Chen, Tui, Kun, Ken, Sun, Chien* as you picture each trigram in the pakua on your abdomen. Then spiral your fingers in the middle and chant *Tai Chi, Tai Chi, Tai Chi,* until you feel the fire and a whole universe spiraling inside of you.

13. Collect energy at your navel and do Chi Self-Massage.

☯ Facial Pakua/Universal Pakua
(Pages 78–86)

As in the previous exercise, you will chant the name of each trigram, then its lines, then the name again. Use your hands and mind to create the expansion of the yang lines and the contraction of the yin lines.

1. Activate the three fires and open the three tan tiens to the six directions.

2. Activate Kan (water) on the bridge of your nose. Chant the *yin, yang, yin* lines as you inscribe them on your face. Picture the trigram on your face, then project it out into the universe. When this ocean energy returns to you, place the trigram in your abdomen.

3. Activate Li (fire) in the middle of your forehead as above, chanting the lines and projecting the symbol out into the cosmos. Then

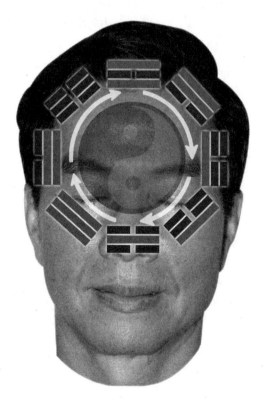

Facial pakua

activate Chen (thunder) at the left temple and Tui (lake) at the right temple, chanting the lines and projecting the symbols out. Place the symbols in your abdominal pakua when they return.

4. Activate Kun (earth) on the upper right eyebrow, Ken (mountain) on the lower left cheekbone, Sun (wind) on the upper left eyebrow, and Chien (heaven) on the lower right cheekbone using the same steps described above.

5. Chant the Tai Chi symbol and spiral it faster and faster, pulling the 8 trigram energies into the center. Connect it to the Crystal Room at the center of your brain and to the center of the lower pakua. Draw all of your senses into the center of this facial pakua, then bring this energy down to the center of the abdominal pakua.

6. Chant *Kan, Li, Chen, Tui, Kun, Ken, Sun, Chien*, touching the trigrams on your abdomen and visualizing the symbols as you chant them. Then spiral the Tai Chi symbol at the center, letting it pull the energies in. Repeat this process for the facial pakua, pulling the energy of your senses into the center.

7. Chant *yin yang, yin yang, yin yang* as you contract and expand your breath and body, then chant *Tai Chi, Tai Chi, Tai Chi.*

8. Chant *Kan* and its lines again, projecting them out into the cosmos. Begin yin yang breathing: as you inhale, let yin contract with bright violet light; as you exhale, let yang expand with bright red light. Continue this breathing until the Kan returns to you and reinforces the kua in your abdomen. Repeat for the other seven trigrams.

9. Picture the pakua in the universe as you chant all the names again. Rest. Feel the universal pakua covering you, breathing and pulsing together with the pakuas in your body. Draw the energy back into your lower pakua, then rest, concentrate, and condense all of the energies in the cauldron.

10. Collect energy at the navel. Do Chi Self-Massage.

COSMIC FUSION

The Creation Cycle (Virtues)

(Pages 135–40)

1. Do the first Fusion formula, forming the four pakuas and the pearl. (See pages 98–99 in level two.)

2. Activate the compassion fire and multi-orgasmic energy and combine them to connect with the universe. Form the pearl by fusing energy inside the body with the universal energy and spiraling them in the cauldron. Bring the pearl down to the perineum.

3. Feel the pearl connecting to the kidneys and their energy of gentleness. Bring the pearl to the kidneys and add their gentle, calm, cool, blue energy to it. Return the pearl to the kidneys' collection point at the perineum, where all of its energy takes on the virtue energy of gentleness.

4. Direct the pearl to the liver, where it activates and enhances the liver's kindness energy. Feel the kindness intensify, and circulate its strong, round, soft, green, warm qualities in the liver. Absorb the kindness

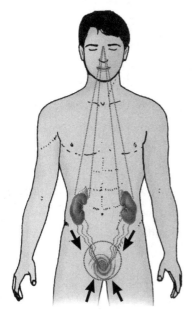

The kidneys' collection point
at the perineum

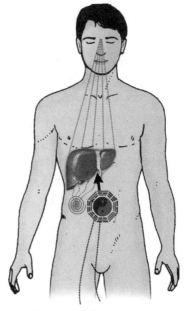

The liver's collection point
on the right of the navel

energy into the pearl, then bring the pearl to the liver's collection point in line with the right nipple at the level of the navel. Here the combination of gentleness and kindness will intensify. Remember to relax and smile.

5. Direct the pearl to the heart, where its energies—especially the kindness energy—activate the heart's love, honor, and joy. Circulate the virtues of the heart, feeling warmth and openness in the chest as the pearl absorbs the deep, calm, red, open energy of the heart.* Bring the pearl to the heart's collection point behind the sternum where it can blend the heart's joy with the gentleness and kindness energies.

6. Bring the pearl to the spleen/pancreas, where its blended energies now activate the spleen's virtues of fairness and openness. Let the pearl absorb the spleen's expansive, clean, dry, yellow, soft energies. Direct the pearl to the spleen's collection point behind the navel, where the fairness and openness energies blend with the virtue energies already present in the pearl.

7. Bring the pearl to the lungs, splitting it in two so that one can circulate in each lung, activating the courage and righteousness there. Let the uplifted, pure white energy of the lungs be absorbed into the pearls, then bring them to the lungs' collection point in line with the left nipple at the level of the navel. Let the pearls blend the righteous energy of the lungs with the energies of kindness, gentleness, honor and respect, and fairness that are already blended there.

8. Direct the two pearls to the kidneys, where their energies enhance the energy of gentleness. Repeat the creation cycle (steps 3–8) 2 more times. In the third cycle move the pearl from collection point to collection point without going to each organ first.

9. Notice the refined quality of your energy, and fuse all the virtue energies into compassion energy. When you feel the compassion energy strongly, move it into the perineum and circulate it through the Microcosmic Orbit, letting it shine. Be aware of the loving, comfortable energies the pearl bestows as it fills the organs with life-force energy. Move the pearl through the Microcosmic Orbit 9–18 times.

---

*Women should not remain in the heart for too long, as their abundant loving energies can heat up the heart center and become uncomfortable.

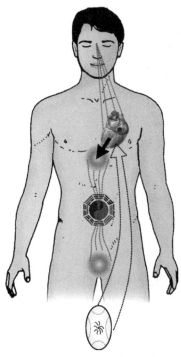

The heart's collection point behind the sternum, blending with kidney energy

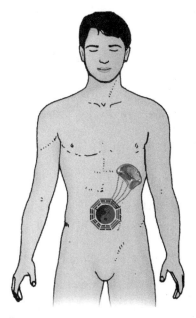

The spleen's collection point behind the navel

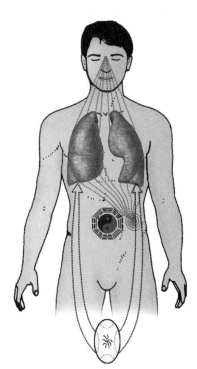

The lungs' collection point on the left of the navel

COSMIC FUSION
Opening the Thrusting Channels

Inhalation during these practices should include many small sips of air, rather than one big breath.

✿ Stage One: Thrusting Channels to the Diaphragm
(Pages 152–59)

1. Begin with the previous exercise, forming a pearl of compassion and bringing it into the perineum.

✿ Left Thrusting Channel to the Diaphragm

2. Inhale through the left nostril, pull up left anus (men add left testicle) and draw the pearl up to the left kidney (women include left ovary). Exhale, letting the pearl drop back down to the left anus/testicle. Practice 9 times.
3. Inhale through the left nostril and draw the pearl up through the left kidney/left ovary to the spleen. Exhale, letting the pearl drop. Practice 9 times.

✿ Middle Thrusting Channel to the Diaphragm

4. Inhale and pull up the middle of the perineum and anus (men add the scrotum). Look up and draw the energy to your prostate or cervix. Relax the eyes and anus, letting the pearl drop back down to the perineum/scrotum. Repeat 8 more times.
5. Inhale, pulling up the anus (men add scrotum). Use the eyes, ears, and nose to draw the energy up to the prostate or cervix, large intestine, small intestine, aorta, and vena cava. Do not thrust beyond the diaphragm. Exhale and feel the Middle Thrusting Channel to this point. Practice 9 times.
6. Repeat steps 4 and 5 above, this time thrusting through the middle organs to the stomach and pancreas. Practice 9 times, then swallow the saliva and rest, feeling the Middle Thrusting Channel up to the diaphragm.

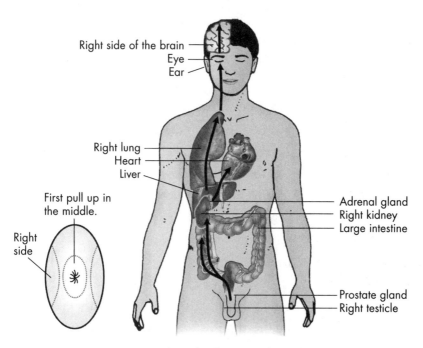

Right side of the brain
Eye
Ear

Right lung
Heart
Liver

First pull up in
the middle.

Right
side

Adrenal gland
Right kidney
Large intestine

Prostate gland
Right testicle

Male Right Thrusting Channel

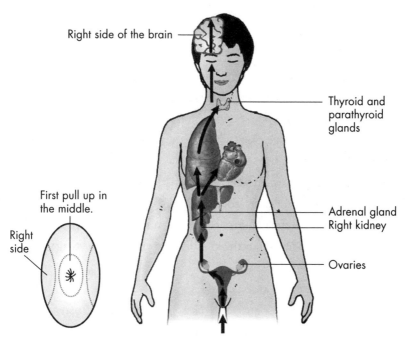

Right side of the brain

Thyroid and
parathyroid
glands

First pull up in
the middle.

Right
side

Adrenal gland
Right kidney

Ovaries

Female Right Thrusting Channel

❀ Right Thrusting Channel to the Diaphragm

7. Repeat steps 2 and 3 on the right side. Use the right eye, ear, and nostril to direct the energy.

❀ Combining All Three Routes

8. Continue to move the pearl through the Thrusting Channels up to the diaphragm in this order: left, middle, right, middle, left, middle, right, middle, left. Continue until the energy is flowing smoothly.
9. Clear the routes with saliva, moving your tongue along your teeth and gums from wisdom tooth to wisdom tooth. Gather the saliva into a ball and swallow it.
10. Circulate the energy in the Microcosmic Orbit, then collect it in the cauldron.

Practice this stage for about 2 weeks, until you can control the energy very well. Practice Spinal Cord Breathing before you progress to the next stage.

❂ Stage Two: Thrusting Channels to the Neck
(Pages 160–61)

1. Left: Practice stage one to below the diaphragm, then return the pearl to the perineum.
2. Bring the pearl up through the left kidney/ovary and the spleen to the left lung, left thyroid, and left parathyroid glands. Hold and exhale, returning the pearl to the perineum. Practice 9 times.
3. Middle: Practice stage one to below the diaphragm, then return the pearl to the perineum.
4. Bring the pearl up from the perineum through the prostate/cervix, intestine, aorta, vena cava, stomach, and pancreas. Continue to direct the pearl up through the heart to the thymus gland and the middle of the neck, thyroid, and parathyroid. Exhale and relax, letting the pearl drop down. Practice 9 times.
5. Right: Repeat steps 1 and 2 on the right side.
6. Combine the three routes and clear with saliva. Finish with the Microcosmic Orbit, then collect the energy in the cauldron.

Practice this stage for 1 or 2 weeks. End by resting and concentrating on all three channels, visualizing the left route as red, the middle as white, and the right route as blue.

Stage Three: Thrusting Channels to the Crown
(Pages 161–66)

1. Left: Practice previous exercises for the Left Thrusting Channel to the neck, then continue thrusting to the left eye, then through the left hemisphere of the brain to the crown. Practice 9 times, then mentally trace the Left Thrusting Channel from perineum to crown.
2. Middle: Repeat practices for the Middle Thrusting Channel to the neck, then continue thrusting to the mid-eyebrow, then up through the pituitary gland to the pineal gland at the crown. Practice 9 times, then mentally trace the whole middle channel.
3. Right: Repeat practices for the Right Thrusting Channel to the neck, then continue thrusting the pearl up to the right eye. Continue thrusting the pearl through the right hemisphere of the brain to the crown. Practice 9 times, then mentally trace the channel.
4. Practice the three Thrusting Channels to the crown 9 times in this sequence: left, middle, right, middle, left, middle, right, middle, and left. Circulate the pearl in the Microcosmic Orbit, feeling the Thrusting Channels joined with the Microcosmic Orbit at the crown and perineum.

Practice this stage for 2 or 3 weeks until you have gained control of the energy. Advanced students may practice extending the three Thrusting Channels above the crown, as shown in *Cosmic Fusion* on pages 164–66.

Stage Four: The Leg Routes of the Thrusting Channels
(Pages 167–69)

1. Form a new pearl by practicing the Fusion and Creation Cycle practices, and bring it into the perineum.
2. Split the pearl in two, and bring the two pearls down the backs of the

legs to the soles of the feet. Absorb earth energy through the soles, then bring the energy up the fronts of the legs to the perineum.

3. Recombine the pearl at the perineum, then run it through the Left Thrusting Channel all the way up to the crown. Extend the pearl 3 inches (7.5 cm) above the crown, then r elax and bring the pearl down to the perineum.

4. Repeat steps 2 and 3, this time running the pearl up the Middle Thrusting Channel through the organs and glands to the crown, then 3 inches above the crown. Relax and return the pearl to the perineum.

5. Repeat steps 2 and 3 again, this time running the pearl all the way up the Right Thrusting Channel to the point about 3 inches above the crown. Return the pearl to the perineum.

🌸 Bringing the Energy into the Ground

6. After you have practiced bringing the pearl down to the soles for a while, practice shooting the energy from the perineum down the backs of the legs and *through* the soles, extending 6–12 inches (15–30 cm) into the ground.

7. Feel a rooting to the earth, then draw the energy up to the soles, up the front of the legs, and into the Thrusting Channels.

🌀 Complete Thrusting Channels Practice

Men and women practice the complete meditation in different ways. Both begin with Fusion, Creation Cycle, and Thrusting Channels practices, then bring the pearl to the perineum.

1. Men: Bring the pearl from the perineum up to and out of the crown, absorbing heavenly energy. Bring the pearl back into the body and let it split in three, continuing down through all three Thrusting Channels down the backs of the legs and into the ground. Absorb earth energy and bring the pearl back into the body, then shoot it out from the toes, around the body, and into the crown. Draw the pearl back into the perineum and repeat 8 more times.

2. Women practice in the reverse: Divide the pearl at the perineum into two, bring it down the backs of the legs into the ground, and absorb earth energy. Bring the energy back into the body, up the front of the legs, and into the perineum. Split the pearl three ways and circulate it through all three Thrusting Channels, up to and out of the crown like a fountain. Let the energy pour out around the body and reenter at the soles of the feet. Repeat 8 more times.

3. Men and women collect energy at the cauldron and practice Chi Self-Massage.

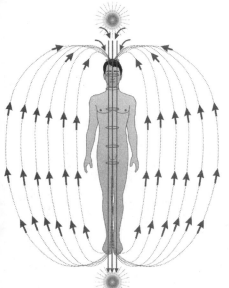

Male Thrusting Channels practice

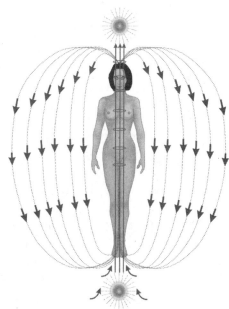

Female Thrusting Channels practice

COSMIC FUSION

Opening the Belt Channels
(Pages 178–86)

As you ascend the Belt Channels, you will circulate the pearl around the body counterclockwise—meaning from the navel to the left side, to the Door of Life, to the right side, and back to the navel. As you descend the Belt Channels you will circulate clockwise—to the right side, Door of Life, left side, navel.

1. Practice the Inner Smile, Fusion of the Five Elements, forming the pakuas and collection points, forming the pearl, and the Creation Cycle. Then send energy through three full Thrusting Channels.

2. Form four pakuas and a pearl, then bring the pearl to the navel. Cir-

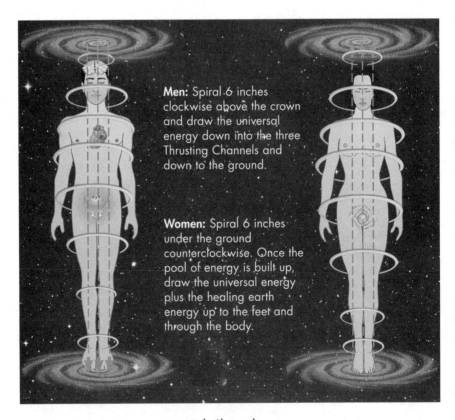

Men: Spiral 6 inches clockwise above the crown and draw the universal energy down into the three Thrusting Channels and down to the ground.

Women: Spiral 6 inches under the ground counterclockwise. Once the pool of energy is built up, draw the universal energy plus the healing earth energy up to the feet and through the body.

Belt Channels

culate the pearl counterclockwise 9 times. Form a cross with the pearl inside the body, connecting the cauldron to the Door of Life and the left pakua to the right.

3. Move the pearl up to the left side of the rib cage, level with the solar plexus. Circulate leftward, through T11 at the back, around the right side, and ending at the solar plexus. Circle 9 times, then create an internal cross, moving the pearl from front to back, and then from left to right.

4. Continue up the left side and circulate 9 times each at the heart center, throat center, mid-eyebrow point, and crown. Form an internal cross with the pearl at each level before moving to the next level.

5. After the crown center, shoot the pearl out through the crown and circle leftward 9 times to form a halo of energy, then form the internal cross.

6. Reverse the direction of energy flow and circle the halo to the right 9 times. Form the internal cross by connecting front to back and the right side to the left side.

7. Bring the pearl in to the right side of the crown and circle rightward 9 times, followed with a cross.

8. Repeat the rightward circles and internal crosses at the mid-eyebrow center, throat center, heart center, solar plexus center, and navel center.

9. From the navel, women bring the pearl down to the right side of the Ovary Palace, 3 inches below the navel. Men bring it down to the right side of the Sperm Palace, 1.5 inches below the navel. Circle rightward 9 times, then trace the internal cross, returning the pearl to the front of the sexual center.

10. Continue to follow the Belt Channels down, circling rightward 9 times and forming internal crosses at the groin, knees, bottoms of the feet, and in the earth below the feet.

11. Reverse direction beneath the earth and circle counterclockwise again 9 times. Form the internal cross connecting front to back and left side to right side.

12. Continue to make leftward circles and crosses at the soles of the feet,

knees, groin, and Ovary Palace/Sperm Palace. Return the pearl to the navel and the cauldron.

🌸 Women Continue Here

1. Bring the pearl to the soles of the feet, then shoot it 6–12 inches into the ground to collect earthly energy. Circle 9 times clockwise, then 9 times counterclockwise.
2. Spiral up through the Belt Channels to the crown, beginning at the left side of each channel and spiraling counterclockwise.
3. Shoot the pearl out of the crown to collect heavenly energy. Circle the energy 9 times counterclockwise, then 9 times clockwise, and bring it back in through the right side of the crown.
4. Continue to spiral the energy clockwise down the Belt Channels to the soles of the feet, then return the pearl to the navel and the cauldron.

🌸 Men Continue Here

1. Bring the pearl to the crown, then shoot it 3–6 inches above the head to collect heavenly energy. Circle the pearl 9 times counterclockwise and 9 times clockwise, then bring it back into the Crown point.
2. Spiral down through the Belt Channels to the soles of the feet, beginning at the right side of each belt and spiraling clockwise.
3. Shoot the pearl 6–12 inches into the ground to collect earthly energy. Circle 9 times clockwise, then 9 times counterclockwise.
4. Return the pearl to the front of the crown, then back down to the navel and the cauldron.

COSMIC FUSION
Advanced Practice Formulas

(Pages 192–97)

⊙ Energy Body/Soul Body

You can form a soul body above the crown of your head, or below the soles of your feet.

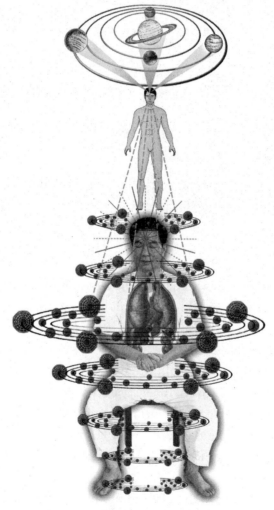

Energy/soul body

1. Begin with the Fusion of the Five Elements practice, then do the Creation Cycle, Thrusting Channel, and Belt Channel practices. Circulate the pearl in the Microcosmic Orbit, then move it to the perineum.

2. Inhale short sips to the navel, heart, and crown while pulling up the anus. Swallow saliva and exhale forcefully to shoot the pearl out of the crown, or down through the soles.

3. Relax the senses and form the soul body.

4. Circulate the pearl in the physical body's Microcosmic Orbit, then open the crown (or soles) and transfer the Mircrocosmic pathway into the soul body. Form another pearl in the physical body and shoot it into the soul body, then circulate the two pearls in both energy bodies together.

5. Extend the Thrusting Channels and then the Belt Channels into the soul body, then spiral all the pakuas around the soul body like a spaceship.

Spirit Body

Be aware of the four pakuas at each energy center and spiral them around the physical body and the energy body.

Stage One

1. Complete the Soul Body practice, leaving the soul body above the crown. Then form another pearl in the cauldron and do the Creation Cycle practice (see pages 187–89 in this book), forming a compassion pearl at the heart. Circulate this pearl in the Microcosmic Orbit and bring it down to the perineum.

2. Inhale in small sips while pulling up the anus and draw the pearl to the navel, heart, and crown. Inhale again and swallow saliva upward, exhaling the pearl into the perineum of the energy body/soul body.

3. Exhale again, sending the pearl to the heart of the soul body, then above the crown of the soul body. Move the pearl up and down 6 feet above the soul body.

4. Condense the pearl and the soul body, bringing both pearls back into the cauldron of the physical body.

Stage Two

5. Repeat steps 1–3 above, and form the spirit body above the energy body.

6. Circulate the pearls in the Microcosmic Orbits of the physical and energy bodies, then copy the Microcosmic Orbit from the energy body into the spirit body. Run all three Microcosmic Orbits together.

7. Extend the Thrusting Channels and then the Belt Channels into the spirit body.

8. Finish by condensing the energy of the soul and spirit bodies into a pearl, which you then pull into the physical body.

9. Collect energy at the cauldron, and practice Chi Self-Massage.

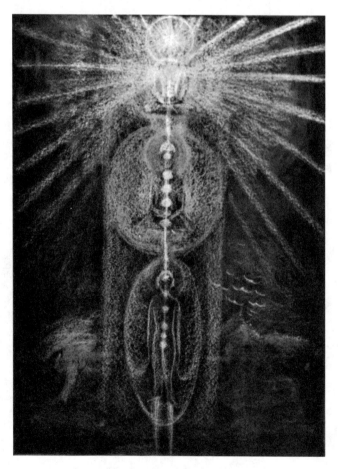

Physical body, energy body, spirit body

THE HEALING ENERGY OF SHARED CONSCIOUSNESS

(Pages 52–57)

⟳ Activating the Three Fires (Tan Tien, Kidney, and Heart)

1. Empty your mind down to lower tan tien.
2. Smile down to your tan tien and feel its fire. Move the yang energy of the adrenal glands down to the center of each kidney at the Door of Life, lighting the fire under the sea. Smile down to the heart, creating softness and the fire of love.
3. Make a triangle, connecting these three fires, and fuse the three minds into one mind (Yi). Expand to the six directions.
4. Become aware of your personal star and connect it to your Yi power. Link your personal stars to your energy body and to the universe.

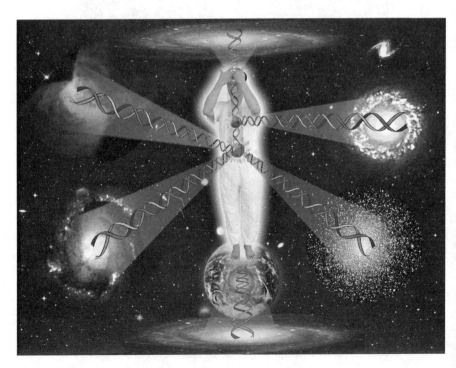

Expanding Yi power to the six directions

⟳ Circle of Fire

1. Visualize a cauldron in the cosmos, burning with fire. Ignite your three fires and expand to the six directions. Create a wand with Yi power and light it from the cauldron fire.
2. Draw a circle of fire about 7 feet (2m) in diameter. Stand in the center facing north, and place a protective animal in each direction. To the north (Blue Tortoise), to the south (Red Pheasant), to the east (Green Dragon), to the west (White Tiger). Above (Yellow Phoenix), and below (Black Tortoise).
3. Create a protective dome of golden chi around you and use an affirmation to connect with universal love: "I am worthy of divine love and protection."

⟳ World Link: Protective Healing Meditation Practice

1. Smile down to your tan tien; direct the heart's mind to the tan tien. Fuse three minds into one mind, Yi, at the mid-eyebrow point and connect with universal energy. Repeat affirmations: "I am at peace in my heart and calm in my center. I am at peace with my family, friends, and community. I am at peace with my enemies and offer them love."
2. Spiral Yi upward through the crown, then into your personal star and whole body. Spiral forest-green healing light down through your community, home, and into your body through the crown. Repeat 3–6 times, then spiral sky-blue ocean-energy light in the same way, repeating 3–6 times.
3. Gather electric violet energy from the Big Dipper and North Star, spiraling them down to fill all your cells and your energy body. Repeat 6 times.
4. Fill the brain with violet light as you affirm: "Let all sickness go away and let the brain be at its very best." Repeat this step and affirmation for the all the orifices, glands, and organs of your body.
5. Touch above your pubic bone and the midpoints of your femur and humerus, penetrating into the sacrum and bone marrow to activate red and white blood cells.

6. Touch the sternum, projecting chi into the chest cavity and activating the thymus, thyroid, and parathyroid glands.

7. Recite affirmations to clear any guilt and negative thought patterns. Picture your physical, emotional, mental, and spiritual bodies, affirming health and harmony in all aspects of your being and sending these images out to the universe.

8. Send any questions or problems through your tan tien and heart center to the mid-eyebrow point, then out into the universe. Acknowledge and follow through on any solutions that come to you.

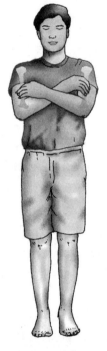

Touch the middle point
of the humerus.

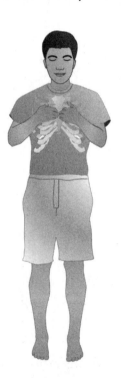

Touch the sternum,
activating the
thymus, thyroid, and
parathyroid glands.

THE HEALING ENERGY OF SHARED CONSCIOUSNESS

Manifestations: Virtuous Mind Power

(Pages 45–50)

Say each command aloud 3 times, followed by the words "Right Now!" Send the commands upward to empty space, then visualize what you want reflecting back. Begin each line with "I am grateful that . . ."

1. (Spirit) "I manifest and feel the glory of my God this day."
2. (Physical) "I am perfectly healthy weighing ____ lbs, seeing with 20/20 vision, possessing a strong body, and feeling balanced (pH)."
3. (Financial) "I accept and feel my fabulous wealth potential generating $_____ of passive income per month."

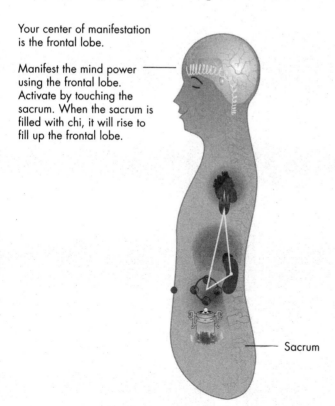

Your center of manifestation is the frontal lobe.

Manifest the mind power using the frontal lobe. Activate by touching the sacrum. When the sacrum is filled with chi, it will rise to fill up the frontal lobe.

Sacrum

Mind power and manifestation

Mid-eyebrow —

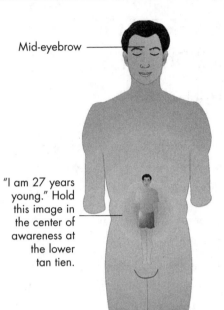

"I am 27 years young." Hold this image in the center of awareness at the lower tan tien.

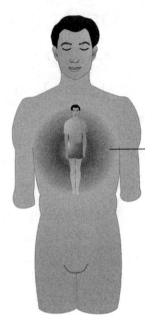

Move up to the center of consciousnes the middle tan tien.

The center of manifestation is the frontal lobe, the upper tan tien.

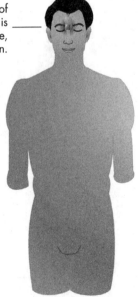

Manifesting on the physical level

4. (Emotional) "I own this day the truth of my past emotions from my birth, youth, and adulthood, and can express and feel all my desires with positive intentions."

5. (Knowledge) "I possess and feel all universal knowledge within my cells' DNA and can open it up on command to answer any questions I have."

6. (Heart) "I fill my heart with radiant joy in a merry way, feeling away all unneeded thoughts, opening my heart, and feeling presence with the power of *Now*."

7. (Age) "I am forever and *feel* _____ years young."

8. (Wisdom) "I accomplish and *feel* every intention to wisdom with everything/anything I do."

9. "So be it: When I feel light there is no darkness."

10. "I fill my body with a golden light, opening my endocrine system and feeling my hormones build, maintain, and sustain my physical immortality."

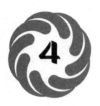

Level Four

Level Four consists of the basic practices of the Universal Healing Tao system that appear in the following titles from Destiny Books: *Energy Balance through the Tao, Tan Tien Chi Kung, Simple Chi Kung, Cosmic Detox, Tendon Nei Kung, Cosmic Astrology,* and *Fusion of the Eight Psychic Channels.*

The practices in this chapter provide students with guidance and exercises for strengthening the physical body, cultivating the yin, and further developing the energy body.

ENERGY BALANCE THROUGH THE TAO

Theory: *Energy Balance through the Tao* presents the Universal Healing Tao's Tao Yin practice. Tao Yin focuses on growing the tendons, relaxing the psoas muscle and the diaphragm, developing strength and flexibility in the body, releasing toxins through the breath, and training the second brain in the lower tan tien to coordinate and direct these processes. The goal of Tao Yin, as with all Chinese internal arts, is to guide and harmonize chi.

Concept: With the Tao Yin breathing techniques you direct energy to and from specific areas of the body—dark energy out of and bright energy in to the upper and lower abdomen, sacrum, chi belt, lungs, etc. Performed in a lying down position, these exercises start the tendon growing process.

Next, you go through a series of postures (like Knee to Chest, Tiger Stretch, Heel to Groin, etc.) that focus on the psoas and sphincter muscles, and on the joint tendons, growing them with each breath. You move through each posture breathing out the dark energy and breathing in the bright energy as you gently lower, raise, twist, and turn each vertebra of the spine.

Purpose: The exercises known as Tao Yin are used as preventives against symptoms of old age and sickness; they are also used to cure certain diseases, both chronic and acute. They can be used for physical, emotional, and spiritual cultivation. The ultimate goal of practicing these Tao Yin energy-directing exercises is to become soft, pure, responsive, and full of energy—like a child. Although these exercises are surprisingly simple to perform, they are sophisticated and effective in reestablishing the harmony we have lost between ourselves, nature, and the universe.

TAN TIEN CHI KUNG

Theory: Traditionally, Chi Kung is the cultivation of the ability to conduct chi for the purposes of healing. Tan Tien Chi Kung is a form of Chi Kung that particularly focuses on working with the lower tan tien. Tan Tien Chi Kung (also called "second brain Chi Kung") is the art of cultivating and condensing chi in the lower tan tien through the Empty Force breathing practices and the Perineum Power exercises.

Concept: When we get older we lose air pressure and we slowly deflate, just as a tire on your car loses air. The years of wear and tear and gravity cause leakages in the body, and we slowly lose the air pressure that gives our bodies form, structure, and constitution. That's one reason why very old people often look like deflated balloons with little bounce or buoyancy. By activating the Empty Force and Perineum Power with dragon and tiger breathing, you can create and increase the chi pressure in your body.

Purpose: Tan Tien Chi Kung is an effective method of bringing us "down to earth" and opening ourselves to receive the energy of the earth. It also helps us to live from our own center and be proactive instead of reactive. Tan Tien Chi Kung proposes that the source of true happiness and joy lies within our very selves and not anywhere else. The negative energies within and around us, which we may experience as obstacles to our happiness, are the raw material for energy transformation. Through this practice we may learn to accept and appreciate ourselves, others, and the world around us. We learn to see our own negative energies as garbage we can compost, which can then serve to fortify our positive energies and increase our health and longevity.

SIMPLE CHI KUNG

Theory: An integral part of the Universal Tao practice, Simple Chi Kung is a series of revitalizing exercises that develop flexibility, strength, resilience, and suppleness. Through their integrative principles, these exercises create harmony within the body, mind, and spirit. This sense of harmony leads us to discover balance within nature and a way to move freely within the ebb and flow of life's ceaseless current.

The Simple Chi Kung formulas of the Universal Healing Tao begin while you are lying in bed. They awaken the body's organs and joints for your daily meditation, Chi Kung practices, and daily activities.

Concept: With so many forms, it is difficult to decide what to learn and what to practice on a daily basis. This exercise series is intended as a condensed Chi Kung practice that will strengthen your body, mind, and spirit in a simple but powerful way.

Purpose: Simple Chi Kung formulas open up your stiff joints after deep sleep, releasing any tensions or stagnant chi. They also lower your blood pressure, activate your bone marrow and blood circulation, engage your immune, respiratory, and digestive systems, and relax your nerves, thoughts, and any emotional imbalances. The movements of Simple Chi Kung start the cultivating, circulating, clearing, exchanging, transforming, and storing processes of your body as you begin your day. They can also be done throughout the day if you feel you have any blockages, stiffness, tension, or discomfort.

COSMIC DETOX

Theory: The body going through life is like a river winding through a forest. As the river flows through at varying speeds and currents, blockages can occur. Branches and trees sometimes fall in, mud builds up, and animals swim through, leaving waste products behind. These can eventually turn the river into a swamp. The only way to get the water flowing freely again is to clear the branches and other debris out of the way.

In our modern world we live in unnatural environments altered by artificial lighting and chemically polluted water, air, and food. These pollutants cause dysfunction and stagnation in our bodies, particularly blocking our nine openings (the mouth, anus, genitals, two eyes, two ears, two nostrils) and the skin—the largest organ of the body. As we get older, the toxins continue to multiply unless we periodically cleanse ourselves of them. This cleansing is a key component of health and longevity.

Concept: The concept of this practice is first to offer different strategies and techniques for opening up blockages within the body. Once the blockages have been removed, deeper-level cleansing and healing can take place. The detox practices offered here include a 14-day total-body cleanse, self-operated colonic irrigation, and some daily practices.

Purpose: We need systematic processes for cleaning and clearing out the built-up toxins in our bodies or we will drown in them. Furthermore, because our Inner Alchemy practices deal with very subtle energies, even small-scale toxins or blockages can affect our practice dramatically. The Cosmic Detox practices are designed to systematically clear the body of toxins so that it can function with maximal health and sensitivity, and remain healthy indefinitely.

COSMIC ASTROLOGY

Theory: In deep meditation the Taoist sages of old could see the molecular sea in which we live, with its repeated patterns in spiraling motions. The sages could detect certain vibrations in the patterns and discovered that they were similar to the behavior of particular animals in nature. They further discovered that these animals could be combined with the five elements—Metal (rocks and the mountain), Water (rivers and the sea), Wood (trees and the forest), Fire (sun and the stars), and Earth (ground and dirt)—to give each animal different phases depending on a person's time of birth. These observations evolved into Chinese astrology.

Concept: Through the Cosmic Astrology formulas and charts, you will be able to find your animal sign and the element for your year, month, and time. It is a simple and complete way to understand why you do the things you do and how you do them.

Purpose: With clearer understanding of your persona (the cosmic energy patterns that determine your personality) you will discover how you think, react to, perceive, and relate to everything and everyone in the universe—as well as and how they think, react to, perceive, and relate to you. These understandings have been calculated, charted, tested, and evaluated for centuries, and now you can use them to help you guide your Inner Alchemy practices and your subsequent transformations.

TENDON NEI KUNG

Theory: Many people hastily want to connect with the "Source" without properly preparing their body. Tai Chi Chi Kung practitioners know that the tendons are the secret to manifesting great power: they have the ability to absorb energy, stretch like elastic, and release up to 93 percent of the energy they absorb. In addition to their inherent elasticity and strength, tendons also have a fantastic capacity for channeling and storing chi. Tendon Nei Kung, the second level of the Iron Shirt Chi Kung practices, focuses on growing and strengthening our tendons for the benefit of our structure, posture, and personal power.

Concept: The more we develop our tendons, the more we unite and connect our various body parts and allow them to function as a unit. Tendon Nei Kung and Iron Shirt practice makes the tendons supple and strong while also opening up the joints. Raw energy can then be stored in these open spaces in the joints and between the tendons, allowing us to take in more energy. Once this is done, we can start to transform this raw energy into higher creative and spiritual energy.

The ancient Taoists followed the theory that the tendons are directly connected to the heart. When the heart contracts, the tendons lightly contract. When the heart expands, the tendons expand. Therefore a vital step in Tendon Nei Kung practice is to be able to strongly sense the beating of the heart so that we can move to its rhythm when doing the forms.

Purpose: The Tendon Nei Kung forms focus specifically on bringing up Earth Chi, making use of our awareness and certain physical movements to encourage the earth's force to rise up through our bodies, nourishing our tendons. Although regular practice of Tendon Nei Kung may yield a vast number of benefits, the exercise is specifically designed to aid in the growth and strengthening of the tendons.

FUSION OF THE EIGHT PSYCHIC CHANNELS

Theory: The Fusion of the Eight Psychic Channels practice builds upon the Inner Alchemy practices found in *Fusion of the Five Elements* and *Cosmic Fusion*. All of these fusion practices focus on clearing the various energy pathways in the body and are prerequisites for the practice of the Immortal Tao. The opening of the psychic channels enables practitioners to balance and regulate energy flows throughout the body and to offer healing energy to Earth as well.

Concept: In this final section of the Fusion practice, the eight psychic channels open the meridian lines of body, beginning with the yang and yin sides of the Regulator and Bridge Channels, then opening up the spine from front to back, up and down, and right to left with Spinal Cord Cutting, Microcosmic, and Aura formulas. Once these formulas are completed you move to open up the crown, five senses, and the heart with drilling and cutting techniques, then seal any energy leaks and protect the body with the final fusion formula—Sealing the Aura. As the sacred energy works into your entire being, it will free your mind from all stresses so that you can see life clearly and be deeply grateful for the life you are able to enjoy.

Purpose: Focusing on the true nature of your spirit will cut away past stresses and misconceptions about life, clearing more room for your divine nature to shine through. When the sacred energy starts pouring out of your entire being into the surrounding environment, the energy will get stronger, pulling you more deeply into beautiful and divine energy. The inner result will be a constant state of strong energy cultivation, eventually resulting in an even higher state of deep relaxation. At this point your energy will be strong enough to achieve any vision you desire, as long as it is aligned with the desires of your spirit. That alignment will naturally allow the energy to keep growing, circulating, and refining, in a continuous cycle that will bring out your highest potential.

ENERGY BALANCE THROUGH THE TAO

Tao Yin Foundations and Exercises for the Spine, Psoas, and Ring Muscles

Full-Body Breathing
(Pages 50–58)

During this exercise, inhale golden light as you smile to your lungs. Draw that light into your body with your breath. When you exhale, expel a cloudy gray color from your body and your lungs.

1. Lie on your back with your legs extended and slightly apart. Place your hands on your navel, right hand over left. Take a few deep breaths, then inhale golden light as you expand your abdomen. Exhale comfortably, guiding the cloudy gray energy out of your body. Continue this breathing for 1 minute or more.

2. Place your hands on your lower abdomen—right hand on your right side and left hand on your left side. Breathe into your lower abdomen as directed above for 1 minute or more, exhaling the cloudy gray energy.

3. Place your hands on your upper abdomen (below the rib cage) and breathe as above.

4. Place your palms on your groin area (inside of each hip) and breathe as above, exhaling down through your legs and out through the soles of your feet and toes.

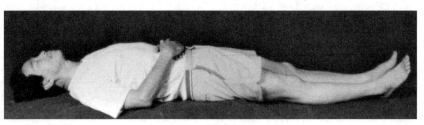

Breathing into the abdomen

5. Bring your right knee up, keeping the foot flat on the floor. Rotate your hips slightly to the left and put your right hand on your sacrum. Put your left hand at the base of your skull. Inhale golden light into your entire spine, exhaling out a cloudy gray color. Continue for 1–2 minutes.

6. Extend your legs again and cross your arms, placing your right palm on your left lower rib cage and your right palm over the right lower rib cage. Breathe as above, into and out of the diaphragm.

7. Keeping your arms crossed, place each palm under the opposite armpit. Inhale golden light into your lungs, imagining that the palms also are inhaling. Exhale the cloudy gray color. Breathe for 2 minutes.

8. Uncross your arms and place your right palm on your upper ribs—under your right collarbone—and your left hand under the left collarbone. Breathe as above into your upper lungs.

9. Place your right palm on the left side of your neck and the left palm on the right side of your neck. Breathe as above, inhaling energy from the bottom to the top of your body.

10. Place your hands on your temples (left hand on left temple, right hand on right), and breathe as above, feeling the temples expanding and contracting as they breathe.

11. Place both hands on the crown of your head and breathe in a steady stream of golden light, exhaling any cloudy gray energy that is still in your body. Feel your crown breathing.

12. Relax, bring your hands to your sides, and breathe normally. Direct chi from your head down to the soles of your feet. Inhale golden light, rais-

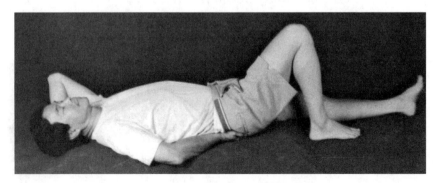

Breathing into the sacrum and Jade Pillow

ing your hands very slowly toward your head, then covering your face softly with both hands. Exhale the cloudy gray color and rub your hands gently down your throat, chest, and abdomen to your groin, then let the energy move down to your heels. Repeat this breath and hand motion several times, bringing your body's energy to an optimal temperature.

The following eight practices to stretch the psoas muscle are done lying on your back.

(Pages 59–82)

❂ River Flows into the Valley

1. Lie on your back, bend your knees, and slide both feet up toward your buttocks, inhaling deeply. (Feet should stay on the floor.)
2. Exhale and push your lumbar spine to the floor by gently lifting your sacrum. Holding this position, raise your chest from the lower thoracic vertebrae, letting the head follow.
3. Inhale and release the sacrum, then return the vertebrae to the mat one by one. Then rest and repeat 2 more times.

❂ Crocodile Lifts Head

1. Lie on your back with legs extended and inhale, bringing your left knee to your chest. Clasp both hands gently over your knee.
2. Lightly tuck your chin and exhale as you press your lumbar spine to the floor and scoop the sacrum up.

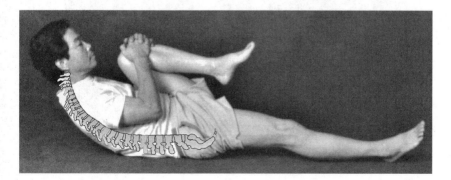

Crocodile Lifts Head

3. Lift your spine beginning with L1 and T12 and moving up. Let the curving of your spine lift your head closer to your knee and hold for a few seconds. Then inhale and release, letting the spine down vertebra by vertebra. Relax and repeat 2 more times.

Monkey Clasps Knees

1. Bring both knees to your chest and clasp them lightly. Tuck your chin and exhale as you press the lumbar spine to the floor and allow the sacrum and thoracic vertebrae to lift up.
2. Press your knees toward your hands as you continue to press the lumbar spine into the mat. Hold without straining for a few seconds, then release and rest. Repeat 2 more times.

Monkey Prays with Elbows (and Counterpose)

1. Lie on your back and bring your knees toward the chest. Extend your arms between the legs, so that the elbows touch the insides of the knees. Reach the arms forward with palms together, lifting the thoracic spine, neck, and head a little bit.
2. Clench your teeth slightly and press the tip of your tongue to the roof of your mouth. Exhale and press the lumbar spine down and raise the sacrum from T12. Using the lumbar muscles (not the thigh muscles),

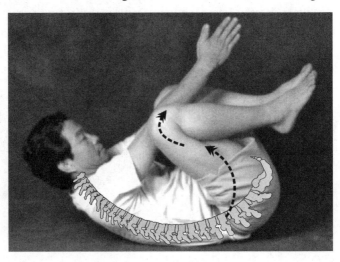

Monkey Prays with Elbows

press your knees toward each other at the same time that you press the elbows outward.

3. Inhale, lowering the body. Then repeat steps 1 and 2 several times. Relax and breathe golden light all the way into your body, exhaling cloudy gray energy.

4. Counterpose: Repeat steps 1–3, this time with the hands clasped around the outsides of the knees. In step 2, press your arms inward and your knees outward.

⟳ Twist Body Like a Snake

1. Lying on your back, bring both knees up, with feet remaining on the floor. Let your knees gently fall to the right.

2. Extend your left arm to the left, palm up, and put your right hand on the left side of the lower tan tien. Turn your head to the left. Breathe golden light in and exhale a cloudy gray color.

3. Hold this position for a few minutes, then return to center and reverse.

⟳ Balanced Bow

1. Lie on your back with legs extended and arms at your sides. Breathe deeply, then press your lumbar spine to the mat and raise your legs slightly, then your upper body.

2. Exhale and stretch your arms toward your feet, raising your legs about 6 inches from the floor. Tuck your chin and raise your head and neck; hold, then release on the inhalation. Repeat.

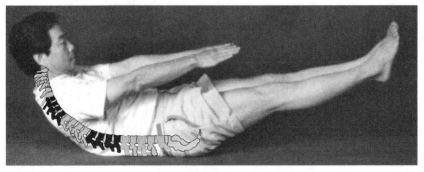

The Bow

☺ Mountain Rises from the Sea

1. Lie on your back with arms at sides, palms down. Bend your knees and slide your feet toward the buttocks. Exhale and tilt the sacrum upward, then L5.
2. One by one, tilt each lumbar vertebra up, then continue with the thoracic vertebrae one at a time, keeping your neck and head flat on the mat as you roll slightly onto your shoulders. Stop when you get to the first cervical vertebra (C7), and just push your body upward.
3. Hold for a few moments, then exhale and come down vertebra by vertebra. Repeat.

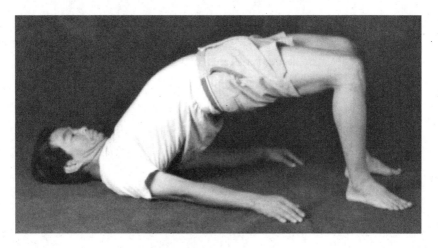

Mountain Rises from the Sea

☺ Cricket Rests on Flower

1. Repeat the previous exercise, but don't stop at C7. Instead, place your palms on the floor over and behind your head, so that your fingers point toward your feet. Roll from the base of your skull to your crown, then push up with your hands and feet to lift your backside off the mat. Only your hands, feet, and crown should touch the mat.
2. Inhale and roll down from top to bottom. Relax and repeat.

⊘ Snake Turns at Wing Point

(Page 83)

The Wing point is on the midline of the back, between T5 and T6.

1. Lie on your back, holding the outside of each shoulder with the opposite hand. Bring your knees up, keeping your feet on the floor. Tuck your chin and exhale as you lift your upper body from the Wing point.
2. Continuing to exhale, twist your upper body and head to the left, lifting only T6–T1 and your head off the mat. Inhale and come back to center, keeping your upper body lifted.
3. Exhale and twist to the right, then inhale and return to center. Relax onto the mat and bring golden light to the Wing point. Repeat 3 times.

⊘ Sphincter Ring (Chi) Muscles

(Pages 94–95)

Lie on your back with your knees bent and feet flat on the floor, palms at your side facing down. With each step below, exhale as you contract and hold the ring muscles, then relax and inhale, keeping your eyes closed.

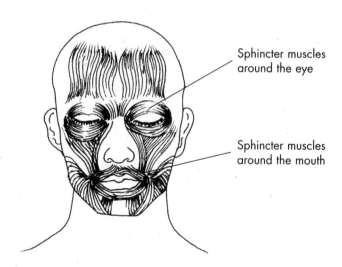

Sphincter muscles around the eye

Sphincter muscles around the mouth

The sphincter muscles of the face and around the eyes and mouth

1. Squeeze your eyes and mouth shut as you exhale: squeeze the area all around your eyes, and pucker your lips tightly, pushing the upper lip toward the nose. Then inhale and relax.

2. Do a series of double contractions of these same muscles, then inhale and relax. Then do a series of multiple rapid contractions, then inhale and relax. Each round should last 5–10 seconds.

3. Repeat steps 1 and 2, this time adding hand and foot contractions, squeezing your fists and the bottoms of your feet. At the same time, press the lumbar spine down and tilt the sacrum up.

4. Exhale and contract the urethral sphincter (as if trying to stop the flow of urine) as you press the lumbar spine down and tilt the sacrum up. Try to focus only on the urethral sphincter, separating it from the anal sphincter. Then inhale and relax. Repeat step 2 with this muscle.

5. Exhale and contract the anal sphincter as you press the lumbar spine down and tilt the sacrum up. Inhale and relax, then repeat step 2 with this muscle.

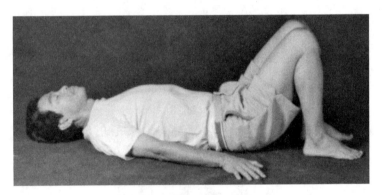

Contracting the ring muscles

6. Contract the front and rear sphincters simultaneously, along with the lumbar and sacrum movements. Inhale and relax, then repeat step 2 with these muscles.

7. Contract the eyes, mouth, hands, feet, and front and rear sphincters simultaneously, along with the lumbar and sacrum movements. Inhale and relax, then repeat step 2 with these muscles. Then rest and smile.

ENERGY BALANCE THROUGH THE TAO

Tao Yin Exercises for Developing Mind-Eye-Heart Power and Growing the Tendons

(Pages 113–20)

❂ Peacock Looks at Its Tail

1. Lie face down with your palms on the floor at mid-chest level. Push your arms to raise your upper body, and slide your right knee forward under your chest. Adjust hands to line up with the right knee. Tuck your chin and lower your spine (from the lumbar vertebrae upward) onto your right thigh. Lean toward your right side, then slowly twist the vertebrae up and toward the right. When the lumbars are fully rotated, twist the thoracics, then your shoulders, neck, and head to look at your right heel. Then return to center, again from the tan tien/lumbar vertebrae upward.

2. Repeat 2 more times, then reverse sides, with your left knee under the body and rotating toward the left. Rotate to the left 3 times.

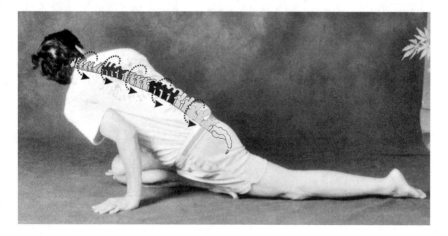

Peacock Looks at Its Tail

☢ Monkey Rotates Spine to Leg (Out)

1. Sit erect with your right leg stretched in front of you and your left knee bent so that the sole of your left foot lies flat against the inside of your right thigh, near the groin. Place your hands on the outside of the right leg: right hand just above the knee and left hand just below it. Tuck your chin and bend forward (from the lumbar vertebrae upward) over your right leg. In this position, rotate your spine toward the right, ending with your neck and head. Return to center, then rock on your sitz bones.

2. Repeat this exercise with your hands on your mid-calf, then again with your hands near your ankle. Then switch legs and rotate toward the left for a total of 3 times.

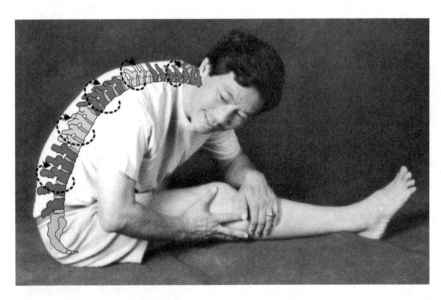

Monkey Rotates Spine to Leg (Out)

✿ Pull Bow and Shoot the Arrow

(Pages 168–71)

1. Sit cross-legged with a tall spine. Fold the pinkie, ring, and middle fingers of both hands: hold the right hand a few inches in front of the sternum with the thumb pointing out and the left hand extended with the palm facing to the left.
2. Bend forward from the lower lumbar vertebrae, then begin to rotate your spine to the left, continuing from the lumbar vertebrae all the way up to the neck and head. Bring your right shoulder a little bit forward and the left shoulder a little bit back.
3. Inhale and pull your left arm back at the same time that you pull your right arm back, as if drawing a bow. Bring your scapulae together to open the chest, then exhale and release.
4. Repeat on the right side, then rest.

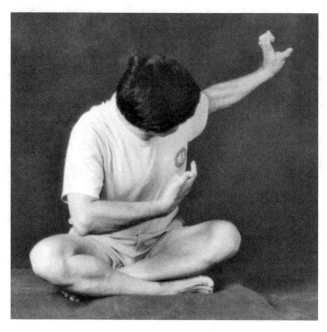

Pull Bow and Shoot the Arrow

❷ Bamboo Swinging in the Wind

(Pages 172–74)

1. Sit with both knees bent: the left leg in front of you with its sole against the right thigh, and the right leg bent behind you with the heel near the buttocks. Hold each ankle with the same-side hand.

2. Rotate only the lumbar spine to the left, so you are over the left leg, then tuck your chin and exhale, bending forward over the left leg.

3. Continuing to exhale, move your torso as far to the left as possible (moving from the lumbar spine). Use your hands to help with the movement. Now rotate your spine to the right, from the lumbars up through the neck and head, again helping with your hands. Hold for a moment, then inhale and release back to center.

4. Repeat this twist 2 more times, then switch legs and twist to the other side 3 times.

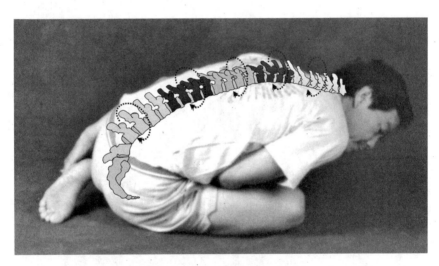

Bamboo Swinging in the Wind
to the right

TAN TIEN CHI KUNG

Empty Force Breath (Dragon and Tiger)
(Pages 73–78)

1. Stand with feet parallel and shoulder-width apart. Put your hands on the Chi Hai (below navel) and breathe deeply. Inhale, then exhale as you flatten and contract the abdomen, pressing in with your fingers.

2. Inhale a half-breath as you make the dragon sound: a high-pitched *hummmmm*. Feel a pressure/sucking sensation in the abdomen and throat. Hold your breath as you pull up the anus, perineum, and sexual organs and expand the abdomen, building pressure in the Chi Hai.

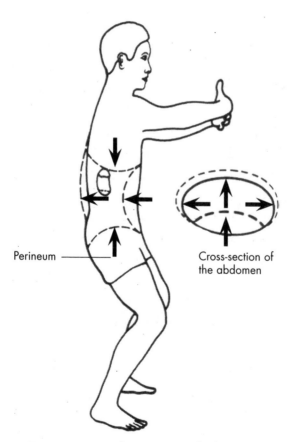

Perineum

Cross-section of
the abdomen

Empty Force Breath: contracting the lower abdomen

3. Exhale with a tiger sound: a low-pitched growling *hummmmm,* as you push the chi pressure down into your lower abdomen. Hold the breath out and laugh softly inside, feeling the Chi Hai vibrate.

Empty Force Exercises
(Pages 79–105)

1. Bladder area: Stand with feet parallel and shoulder-width apart. Maintain awareness at the perineum and the front, back, and middle parts of the anus, as well as at the uterus or prostate.
2. Place your hands on the Chi Hai and breathe, then exhale and contract the abdomen, pushing in with your fingers. Hold the breath out as you pull your abdomen up and in.
3. Inhale one-third of a breath as you make the high-pitched dragon sound; contract and pull up your anus at the same time. Feel vacuum pressure in the abdomen and throat.
4. Inhale the second third of breath as you contract and pull up the front part of the anus and the sexual organs toward the bladder/uterus. Expand your abdomen.
5. Inhale the last third as you continue to pull up the front part of the anus toward the bladder. At the same time, push your lower abdomen out against your fingers. Keep your tongue against your palate and hold the breath in.
6. Exhale with the kidneys' sound, choo-oo-oo-oo, feeling your coccyx turn in and your sacrum pushing out. Laugh softly inside and feel the vibration. Repeat steps 1–6 a few more times, then relax and and smile.
7. Solar plexus: Repeat steps 1–6, this time placing your hands on your solar plexus and contracting your anus and perineum toward the solar plexus.
8. Sides of the tan tien: Repeat steps 1–6 again, this time placing your fingers on the left and right sides of the lower tan tien. Your awareness and contractions will be on the left and right sides of the anus, as well as the perineum.

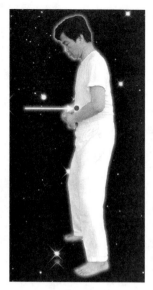
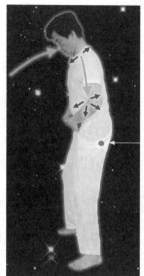
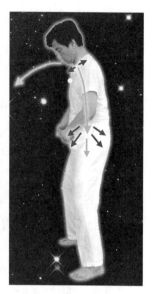

| Contract the abdomen. | Feel the vacuum pressure. | Exhale with the kidneys' sound. |

9. Repeat these steps for each of the following areas: the sides of the body, the kidneys, Ming Men, and the chest.

10. Repeat for the whole lower tan tien, pulling the front, left, and right sides of the anus up toward the front, left, and right sides of the abdomen, then inhaling again and pulling the left, right, and back sides of the anus up toward the left and right kidneys and the Door of Life.

⊙ Tan Tien Chi Kung Warm-Up
(Pages 109–11)

1. Stand with feet shoulder-width apart, toes pointed slightly inward. With both hands, rub your sacrum, then move it back and forth.

2. With hands at your sides, gently spiral your knees and ankles outward. Exhale, pressing your heels into the ground, keeping the big toes slightly inward. Press your legs firmly into the earth, keeping the bones rotated outward.

3. Feel the hip bones separating from the sacrum. At the same time, push the sacrum back and tuck the coccyx in.

TAN TIEN CHI KUNG

⊙ Animal Postures

(Pages 112–50)

Begin each posture with feet parallel and shoulder-width apart, and your arms at your sides. Begin by inhaling with the dragon sound as you pull up the anus and perineum, then exhaling with the tiger sound.

End each posture with the ending exercise, labeled step 2 below.

1. **Rabbit (front tan tien):** Inhale and raise your arms above your head with wrists bent downward. Exhale quickly with the tiger sound, pulling the anus up and widening your nostrils. Sink down, then press the palms down and out, pushing chi pressure into the front of the lower tan tien with the tiger sound. Repeat several times.

2. **Ending exercise:** Stand with your feet together and scoop energy up as you inhale. Turn palms downward and pour the energy over the body and into the navel and lower tan tien, focusing on the Door of Life. Move hands to thighs and absorb chi into the thigh bones, then glide hands down your legs as you squat down. Sink through the earth and feel universal energy spiraling. Put your hands on your feet

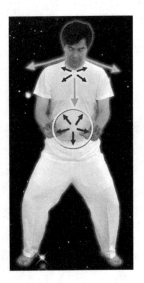

Rabbit

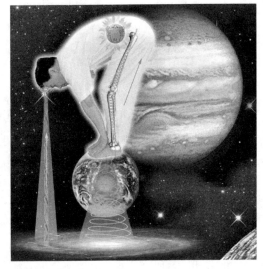

Ending exercise

and lift your tailbone—drawing chi into your body—until your legs are straight. Squat and stand 3–9 times, then press energy with your fingers into your shinbones, coccyx, sacrum, sexual center, and Door of Life. Bring hands to navel and store the energy.

3. **Crane (sides of the tan tien):** Inhale (dragon sound) as you pull up the anus and perineum. At the same time, raise your arms above your head and form beaks with both hands. Exhale quickly (tiger sound) as you pull the left and right sides of the anus up more. Sink down and press the palms down to hip level, then out to the sides. With sound, push chi pressure down and out into the left and right sides of the tan tien. Repeat step 2.

4. **Bear (back lower tan tien, and back):** Inhale (dragon sound) while pulling up the anus and perineum. Raise hands to scoop up chi and pour it down. Exhale with tiger sound, pulling up the back part of the anus a bit more. Sink down, and press the hands down. Twist the ulna and radius bones in opposite directions, then the ankles and knees. Round your shoulders and expand your back. Breathe dragon and tiger breaths, then suck in and out without breathing to increase pressure. Inhale, turn palms up and out, and raise them up to scoop and pour chi. Lower hands to the navel and rest. Repeat step 2.

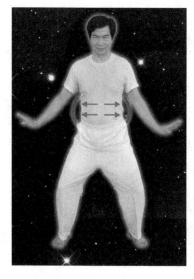 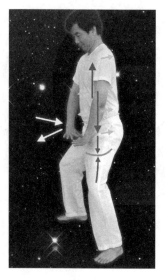

Crane   Bear

5. **Swallow (sides of the tan tien):** Stand in Embracing the Tree posture and inhale (dragon sound), pulling up the anus and perineum, then exhale (tiger sound). Let chi pull you to the left (from the lumbar vertebrae), then inhale and push chi down into the left side of the tan tien, keeping the anus contracted. Feel your left leg pushing into the earth and the force coming up from the earth. Continue dragon and tiger breaths to expand the pressure, then rotate back to the middle. Repeat breath and legs in the middle, then to the right side, then back to the center. Repeat step 2.

6. **Dragon (sides of the tan tien):** Inhale and pull up the anus, then exhale quickly. Let chi pull you to the left, and push chi down into the left side, keeping the anus contracted. Expand pressure with dragon and tiger breaths, then exhale quickly, pulling up the left side of the anus as you thrust the right fist downward along the left thigh. Repeat to the middle (with both fists) and to the right (with left fist). Repeat step 2.

7. **Eagle (whole tan tien):** Raise your arms above your head as you inhale, spreading your fingers and rolling your eyes upward. Exhale with the tiger sound, pulling up the anus even more and pressing chi into the tan tien. Repeat 3–6 times, then do step 2.

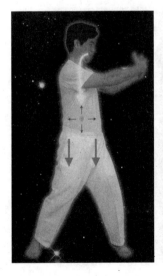 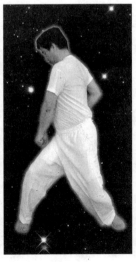 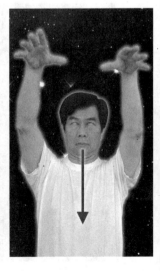

Swallow   Dragon   Eagle

8. **Monkey (lower tan tien):** Stand with your palms in front of the kua. Inhale (dragon sound) and pull up. Feel the vacuum and raise your hands above your head with palms open. Exhale (tiger sound) and squat down from the kua, pushing chi pressure into the lower tan tien. Swing your arms down and backward, then up again. Continue swinging arms as you gather the Earth Chi into your palms and bones. Inhale and rise up with arms up and palms open. Repeat 3–6 times, then do step 2.

9. **Elephant (tan tien left and right sides):** Inhale and pull up, expanding the low abdomen and throat with chi pressure as you hook your thumbs and raise your arms above your head. Turn hips to the left, then exhale and pull up the left side of the anus while pressing chi into the tan tien. Turn hips to center and swing your joined arms down, then back and forth—gathering Earth Chi. Inhale and rise up with arms raised, scooping the Earth Chi up. Repeat to right side, then repeat whole exercise 3 times. Do step 2.

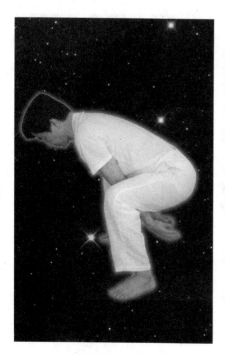

Monkey

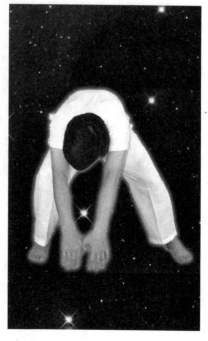

Elephant

10. **Rhinoceros (tan tien left and right sides):** Inhale and pull up, expanding the low abdomen and throat with chi pressure. Step your left foot forward as you rotate your right foot 45 degrees. Hold the back of your right hand in front of your forehead as you stretch the left arm forward, palm down. Inhale, pull up the left side of the anus, and sink down. Rotate waist and upper body to the left without moving the hips. Exhale (tiger) as you press chi into the left side of the lower tan tien and press the left leg into the ground. Repeat dragon and tiger breaths to build up pressure, then release and return to center. Repeat to the right side, then do step 2.

11. **Horse (solar plexus):** Inhale and pull up as you raise your arms above your head and suck in the upper abdomen toward your back. Pull in navel to touch the spine. Sink down and press the arms down with force as you exhale the horse sound—*Ho*—and push out your abdomen. Repeat horse sound with arm movement 3–6 times, then do step 2.

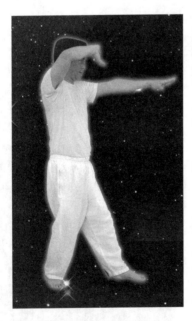

Rhinoceros

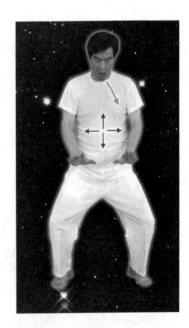

Horse

12. **Bull (back of tan tien):** Inhale and pull up, expanding the low abdomen and throat with chi pressure. Step your right foot forward as you rotate your left foot 45 degrees. Stretch your arms forward with palms down, then sink down, inhale, and pull up. Rotate wrists to scoop up chi on the left and right as you press down into both legs. Spiral the hands under the armpits until the palms face you. Exhale (tiger) as you pull up the front of the anus and press chi down into the lower abdomen. Spiral the palms outward and push your hands forward, pushing energy into the fingertips as you press the Abdominal Chi into your legs. Feel earth energy rise in your legs as you pull up the front and back of the anus, then draw energy into your spine by rounding the scapulae and sacrum and sinking the chest. Repeat the whole exercise in this position, then switch foot positions and repeat entire sequence. Finish with the ending exercise (step 2).

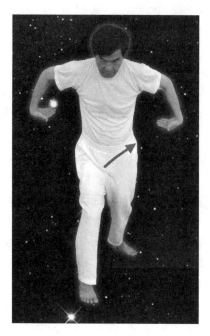

Bull

SIMPLE CHI KUNG

(Pages 61–89)

⚙ Opening the Joints

Stand with your feet shoulder-width apart, knees slightly bent.

1. **Bouncing:** Relax your body and bounce on the floor without any tension. Let your arms hang loosely at your sides and gently vibrate all the joints.

2. **Foot and hand kicking:** Draw up one leg and the opposite arm, then kick out your leg, letting go of any tension or pain. Repeat 30–60 times, then switch sides and repeat.

3. **Knee rotations:** Bring your feet together and bend your knees, placing your palms over your kneecaps. Rotate your knees counterclockwise 3–4 times, then repeat in a clockwise direction.

4. **Hip rotations:** Stand with feet slightly wider than shoulder-width apart and your hands on your hips. Bring your hips forward and rotate them in a large clockwise circle, then tilt them backward and rotate counterclockwise. Repeat these circles 8 more times, then switch directions, rotating counterclockwise when forward and clockwise when backward.

5. **Sacrum:** Place both hands over the sacrum and rotate it 36 times in each direction.

6. **Waist loosening:** Stand with feet slightly wider than shoulder-width apart and arms hanging loosely at your side. Turn your hips side to side and let your arms swing naturally. Relax your spine and let the lumbar vertebrae begin to rotate from the hips, then the thoracic vertebrae, then the cervical vertebrae and shoulders.

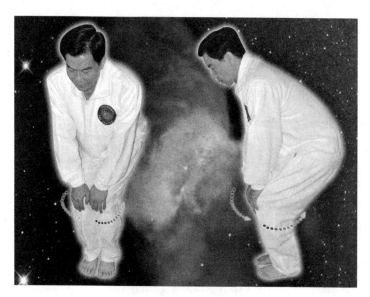

Knee rotations

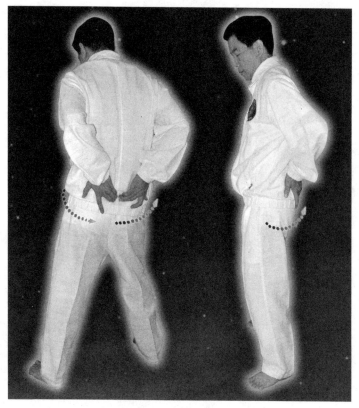

Rotating the sacrum

⊙ Windmill Exercise: Opening the Spinal Joints

1. **Outer front extension:** Stand with feet slightly wider than shoulder-width apart. Hook your thumbs together, keeping your hands close to your body. Inhale and raise your arms with fingers pointing up, extending your spine backward. Exhale slowly and bend forward vertebra by vertebra, keeping your head between your arms. Slowly straighten up, again vertebra by vertebra, leaving your head and arms hanging until the end. Repeat 3 times.

2. **Inner front extension:** Stand wide as above and point your fingertips downward, slowly lowering your arms, then your torso, vertebra by vertebra, until you are completely bent over. Straighten slowly with your head between your arms. When you are completely upright, bring your hands over your head. Repeat 3 times.

3. **Left outer extension:** In the wide stance with your arms overhead, twist your torso to the left, pivoting on your feet. Stretch forward and down toward your left foot. Circle back up on the right side until you are upright with arms overhead. Repeat 3 times.

4. **Right outer extension:** Repeat step 3, but twist and bend to the right, circling back up on the left. Finish by unhooking your thumbs and floating arms down.

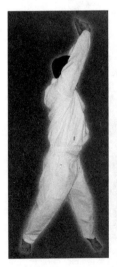 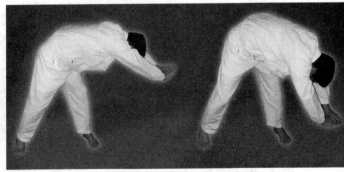

Windmill: left outer extension

🌀 Hand and Wrist Stretches

In these stretches, one arm at a time is active, while the passive arm receives the stretch.

1. **Flexion:** With your active arm, lift the passive wrist to the level of the sternum, then flex the wrist by pushing the hand toward the inside of the arm. Repeat a few times, then switch sides.

2. **Internal rotation:** With the palm of your passive hand in front of your face, wrap your active hand around the back of it, placing the active hand's thumb between the little finger and ring finger while the active fingers wrap around the passive wrist. Rotate the passive wrist by pushing your active thumb toward you as you pull your active fingers backward, pulling the passive wrist. Repeat a few times, then switch sides.

3. **External rotation:** Stand with arms outstretched, palms facing each other. Turn your passive hand outward and support it with your active hand, letting the whole weight of the elbow and shoulder drop.

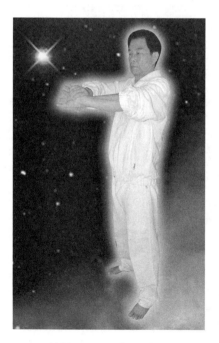

Wrist external rotation

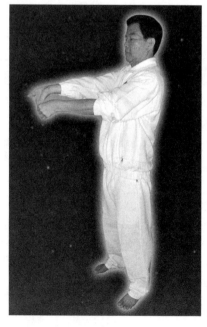

Wrist downward hyperextension

Use your active hand to flex the passive wrist toward your body. Repeat, then switch sides.

4. **Upward hyperextension:** Extend your passive arm forward with palm out and fingers pointing up. Place the palm of your active hand against the fingertips of the passive hand and pull them gently toward you, dropping the passive arm and shoulder to hyperextend the wrist. Then let the active hand lift the passive arm all the way up, feeling the stretch from the fingers to the neck. Repeat and switch sides.

5. **Downward hyperextension:** Extend the passive arm forward with the palm up. Use the active hand to bend the passive fingers downward, hyperextending the fingers, hand, wrist, and arm. Repeat and switch sides.

⊘ Stretching the Neck and Shoulders

1. **Neck:** Let your head drop gently to one side then the other. Next, rotate your neck side to side, looking over each shoulder. Then lift your chin up and down. Repeat this whole sequence 9 times.

2. **Shoulder rotations:** Stand with your feet shoulder-width apart and arms hanging. Bring your shoulders all the way up to your ears, then as far back as possible, then down to resting position. Stretch your arms downward from your fingertips to your spine. Repeat 3 times.

3. **Arms forward:** Stand with your arms extended all the way forward. In this position rotate your shoulders up, back, and down, then stretch your arms from fingertips to spine. Repeat 3 times.

4. **Arms up:** Repeat the shoulder rotations as above, this time with your arms stretched overhead.

5. **Arms to sides:** Repeat the shoulder rotations with your arms stretched out to your sides.

⊘ Opening the Door of Life

1. Stand with feet slightly wider than shoulder-width apart and arms hanging loosely at your sides. Rotate your hips to the left, letting your right arm swing in front of you, raising it to head height (palm facing

out). At the same time, let your left arm swing behind you and place the back of the hand over the Door of Life point.

2. At the end of your rotation, loosen your lower back to extend a little bit more. Extend in this way 3 times, then repeat steps 1 and 2 toward the right. Repeat 9 times on each side.

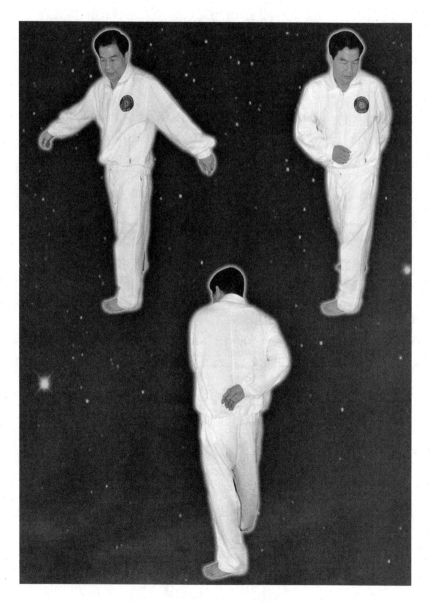

Opening the Door of Life

COSMIC DETOX

Cellular Cleansing

(Pages 47–50)

During this 7–14-day cleanse, you eat no solid foods; instead, you take supplements, drink vegetable broths, and make the following cell-cleansing drinks. The drinks should be mixed separately, and then drunk in succession 5 times each day.

First Drink

Place the following in a jar and shake for 15 seconds, then drink quickly.

2 oz. apple, lemon, or lime juice   8 oz. pure water

1 tablespoon colloidal bentonite   1 teaspoon psyllium

Second Drink

Place these ingredients in a pint jar, then shake and drink.

10 oz. pure water

1 tablespoon apple cider vinegar or other vinegar

1 teaspoon honey or pure maple syrup

Supplements

Follow the schedule below for the correct dosage and timing of the supplements, which should be taken 4 times per day, 1.5 hours after the cleansing drinks.

SUPPLEMENT SCHEDULE (4 times per day)

	Day 1	Day 2	Days 3, 7, & 14
Chlorophyll gel tablets	12	18	24
Vitamin C tablets	200 mg	200 mg	800 mg
Pancreatin tablets	6	6	6
Beet tablets	2	2	2
Dulse tablets	1	1	1
Enzymatic tablets	2	2	2
Niacin tablets	50 mg	100 mg	200 mg
Wheat germ oil tablets	1	1	1

⟳ Self-Operating Colonic System

(Pages 38–43)

Do two colonics per day for 7 days, or one colonic every other day for 2 weeks.

1. Set colonic board hood on toilet and the board on a stool.
2. Hook up tubing to bucket, then fill with warm water and rinse. Check water release. Insert rectal tip into the tube in the board hood. Place the pad on the board and lie on your back, with your buttocks on the hood.
3. Apply rectal gel and insert the rectal tip into your anus.
4. Relax. Release the tube clamp and allow water to flow freely.
5. Massage the left side of your abdomen upward (against the normal direction of flow) toward the bottom of the rib cage. Work through any tender spots. Continue upward, then across the lower border of the rib cage and down the right side of your abdomen.
6. When it becomes necessary to evacuate, relieve your bowels by expelling water. Feces should bypass the tip without pushing it out.
7. Without flushing the toilet, repeat steps 4–6 a few times until the bucket is empty (about 45 minutes). Look at what has come out in the toilet (black/green feces), then flush.

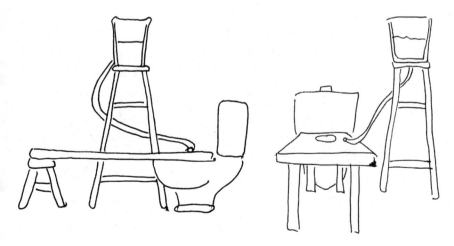

Set-up for an open-ended colonic system that can be self-administered

8. Finish by clamping the tube, removing the tip, and slipping out from the board. Wash the board, then sit on the toilet to defecate. Clean yourself when finished.

9. Collect energy at the navel.

🌀 Implants

The following implants can be placed in the bucket individually or in combinations.

- Chlorophyll liquid concentrate (½ cup of liquid squeezed from green grass)
- Coffee (2 tablespoons ground coffee simmered in 1 quart of water for 15 minutes—strain and add to bucket)
- Garlic (3 cloves blended and strained into bucket)
- Lemon juice (¼ cup strained into bucket)
- Saline (1 tablespoon of sun-dried sea salt into bucket)
- Epsom salts (1 tablespoon dissolved into bucket)
- Glycothymoline (8 ounces per 5 gallons of water)
- Acidophilus (1 quarter of bottle into bucket)

After your colonic series ends, eat only whole fruits and vegetables for 2 days. They can be steamed or cooked into soup. Also take acidophilus twice a day for 2 weeks.

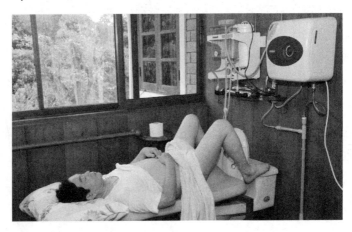

Massaging the abdomen while using a self-operating colonic board

Dry Skin Brushing

(Pages 43–45)

Use a bristle brush or loofah before your morning bath and before bed at night. Gently brush with strokes from outer points of the body to the center. The skin should glow with a pink color; it should not turn red. The total process takes about 3 minutes.

1. Do the Inner Smile meditation, then brush from sole of the right foot up the entire leg to the groin. Use short, quick strokes or long sweeping strokes toward the heart. Use as many strokes as are needed to brush the front, back, and sides of the leg. Repeat for left leg.
2. Brush buttocks, hips, lower back, and abdomen with circular motions.
3. Brush the left arm from the hand up to the shoulder, then circle the left breast. Make sure to brush the top, bottom, and sides of the arm. Repeat for right arm.
4. Brush across the upper back, then down the front, back, and sides of the torso. Cover entire skin surface once.
5. Use a softer brush on the face. Begin in the center of the face and stroke outward. Brush down the sides of the face and neck.

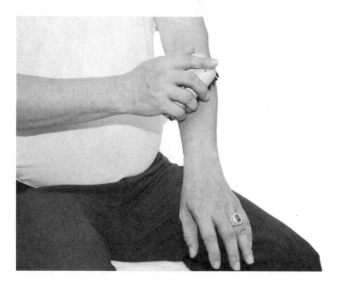

Dry skin brushing

6. To finish, jump into the shower and feel a light, tingling sensation over your body.

7. Clean and dry your body, then collect energy at the navel.

🌀 Solar Bathing
(Pages 45–46)

Expose your entire body to the open air to absorb vitamin D.

1. Use the Inner Smile meditation to smile down to your organs.

2. Lie down naked in a secluded area, absorbing fresh air and the sun's rays for 10 minutes on each side. Work up to 30 minutes on each side by adding 5 minutes each day.

3. Collect energy at the navel. Do the Six Healing Sounds practice.

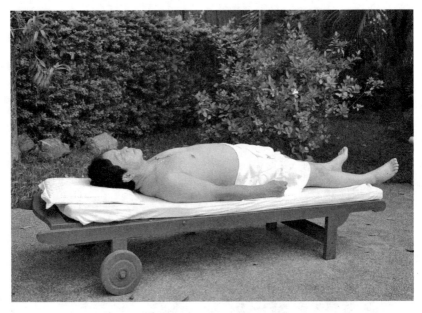

Solar bathing

COSMIC ASTROLOGY

Chinese and Western Combinations
in Theory and Practice
(Pages 213–18)

Comparing your Western sign (month) to your Chinese sign (year) provides a new angle and dimension of your persona. Simply take your regular, familiar astrological sign and match it with the animal sign of the year you were born. If you are a Scorpio and were born in 1948, then you are a Scorpio-Rat. Everybody has a dual nature. Some people are naturally greedy and grasping about money, but the same people can be generous to a fault in emotional ways. The combination of the different aspects of an individual's persona, including sentiment, affection, and phase, could explain this seemingly contradictory behavior. It is true as well in relationships: there are some people you can get along with and care for easily, others who just rub you the wrong way or get on your nerves, and still others who attract and fascinate you. In order to understand your attraction or dislike for a person, you can now use *Cosmic Astrology* to determine his or her persona and apply these discoveries about how to communicate effectively with each individual's internal energy pattern.

This approach attempts to help us understand human behavior within the universe through the marriage of Western and Chinese astrologies. The Chinese have divided time differently from Westerners. Western time is divided into hundred-year-long centuries, while the Chinese have repeating cycles of sixty years. In the West, we divide our centuries into ten decades. The Chinese divide their sixty-year spans into "dozen-cades" or twelve-year periods. In the West, we divide our year up twelve times by its moons. Each month is between twenty-eight and thirty-one days long, and overlaps with one or two of twelve Western astrological signs. Every year the Western cycle begins anew. In the East, each year within the dozen-cade has its own astrological name. At the end of each twelve-year period, the Chinese cycle begins anew.

To review, the twelve Western months have celestial sign names: Aries, Taurus, Gemini, Cancer, Leo, Virgo, Libra, Scorpio, Sagittarius,

Capricorn, Aquarius, and Pisces. The twelve Chinese years have animal sign names: Rat, Buffalo, Tiger, Rabbit, Dragon, Snake, Horse, Ram, Monkey, Rooster, Dog, and Boar. In both cases, the astrological sign name refers to the character of people named under its influence. Though there is a calendar difference with the Western signs and the months of the year, for this application we are using the Western signs as the Chinese animal months. Everyone has a Western "month" sign and a Chinese "year" sign. One sign is complementary to the other, and each Western sign also interacts with its corresponding Chinese sign.

CHINESE ANIMALS, WESTERN SIGNS, AND THEIR ATTRIBUTES

Year	Western Signs	Month	Earthly Branch	Time of Day	Chinese Triad	Secret Allies
Rat	Sagit-tarius	11/23–12/22	Yang Water	11pm–1am	Dragon, Monkey	Snake & Monkey
Buffalo	Capricorn	12/22–01/20	Yin Earth	1am–3am	Snake, Rooster	Horse & Ram
Tiger	Aquarius	01/21–02/19	Yang Wood	3am–5am	Horse, Dog	Dragon & Boar
Rabbit	Pisces	02/20–03/20	Yin Wood	5am–7am	Ram, Boar	Rooster & Dog
Dragon	Aries	03/21–04/20	Yang Earth	7am–9am	Monkey, Rat	Tiger & Boar
Snake	Taurus	04/21–05/21	Yin Fire	9am–11am	Rooster, Buffalo	Rat & Monkey
Horse	Gemini	05/22–06/21	Yang Fire	11am–1pm	Dog, Tiger	Ram & Buffalo
Ram	Cancer	06/22–07/23	Yin Earth	1pm–3pm	Boar, Rabbit	Buffalo & Horse
Monkey	Leo	07/24–08/23	Yang Metal	3pm–5pm	Rat, Dragon	Snake & Rat
Rooster	Virgo	08/24–09/23	Yin Metal	5pm–7pm	Buffalo, Snake	Dog & Ram
Dog	Libra	09/24–10/23	Yang Earth	7pm–9pm	Tiger, Horse	Ram & Rooster
Boar	Scorpio	10/24–11/22	Yin Water	9pm–11pm	Rabbit, Ram	Dragon & Tiger

TENDON NEI KUNG

⊙ Structure, Pressure, Tendon Power
(Pages 37–47)

1. In Iron Shirt stance, lift your toes back and lean slightly forward to lift your heels an inch off the ground. Then press your toes down and rock back onto your heels, transmitting force from the earth to your feet, ankles, and legs.

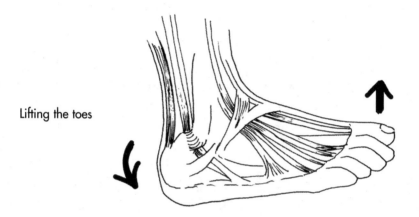

Lifting the toes

2. As you rock forward onto your toes, squeeze your legs slowly from the bottom up.
3. When the force reaches your hip joints, squeeze them together, sending the earth's force upward.
4. Press your psoas muscles from your hips up into the solar plexus and T11.
5. Stretch the spine upward like a wave, expanding each vertebra from bottom to top.
6. Open the scapulae and push T11 toward your back. At the same time, tilt your sacrum by rolling your hips under your body. Feel your feet pressing into the ground.
7. Gently pulse your hands in rhythm with your heartbeat, slightly contracting and expanding your hands as the blood pulses into your fingers.

8. Press your tongue to your palate, connecting the Governing Vessel to the Conception Vessel and activating the cranial pump. Round your shoulders, sink the chest, and tuck your chin, sending earth force through the tendons of the arms and hands. Open your hands as the earth's force reaches your fingers.

9. As your heart contracts and you open your hands, exhale with force by squeezing the lower tan tien like a clenching fist. At the same time, pull up your genitals, close your anus, and pinch your elbow joints to create a slight tension that will torque all the tendons in your body. Then inhale and relax.

Coordinate with Your Heartbeat

10. As your heart expands (diastole), you exhale, rock forward onto your toes, stretch your finger tendons, and pull up your sexual organs.

11. As your heart contracts (systole), you inhale and rock back onto your heels, releasing all tension in the body.

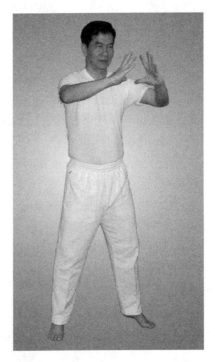

Position when the heart contracts

TENDON NEI KUNG

🌀 The Eight Hand and Arm Positions
(Pages 50–59)

In each of the positions below, you will exhale and inhale as in the previous exercise: rocking back and forth and tightening your tendons in rhythm with your heartbeat to bring the earth's force up through your body.

1. First position: Stand in Iron Shirt stance, with your hands in front of your face, palms inward and fingers pointing toward each other. Exhale and inhale as above. As you exhale, open your scapulae and sink your chest to move your arms forward. At the same time, torque the tendons in your hands, emphasizing the tendons in the middle fingers.

2. Second position: Hold your hands at eye level, with palms slanting toward each other to form a roof shape. Exhale and inhale as above. As your heart expands and you exhale and torque the tendons, let your arm structure move about 1 foot away from your body. Focus on the tendons in your pinkie fingers.

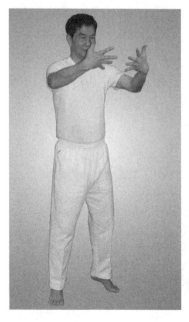
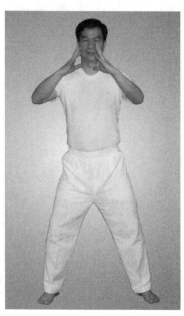

Tendon Nei Kung first position   Tendon Nei Kung second position

3. Third position: Hold your hands at the level of your abdomen with palms facing each other about 8 inches apart. Exhale and inhale as above. When you exhale and torque your tendons from the ankles up, let your arms move forward. At the same time, gently stretch your four fingers forward and your thumbs upward. Focus on the tendons in your thumbs.

4. Fourth position: Hold your hands at abdomen level, with palms facing down. Exhale and inhale as above. When you exhale, move your arms up and out (about 6 inches each way), focusing on the tops of your hands. Feel resistance to the downward force.

5. Fifth position: Stand with your hands about 1.5–2 feet in front of your solar plexus, palms inclined slightly toward each other. Exhale and inhale as above. When you exhale and torque your tendons, move your arms about a foot away from your body. Direct your focus to your pinkie fingers.

6. Sixth position: Hold your hands at shoulder level about a foot from your body, with palms facing your chest and your elbows down and

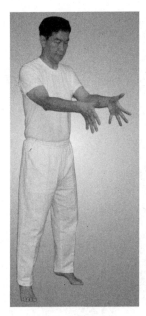

Tendon Nei Kung
third position

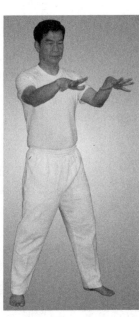

Tendon Nei Kung
fourth position

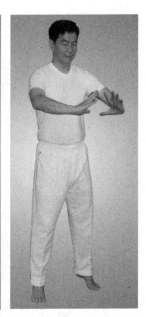

Tendon Nei Kung
fifth position

relaxed. Exhale and inhale as above. As you exhale, let your arms move about 6 inches forward, up, and out, with animated movements. Bring your awareness to your spine and its whiplike motions, feeling it fill with the earth's force.

7. Seventh position: Hold your hands at waist level, with palms facing up and fingers pointing toward each other like a basket. Exhale and inhale as above. As you exhale and torque your tendons, move your arms forward and up about 1 foot. Direct awareness to your spine, feeling it charging with the earth's force.

8. Eighth position: Bend your knees enough to hold your hands a few inches in front of them, with palms facing up. (Keep your back straight.) Exhale and inhale as above. As you exhale and torque your tendons, straighten your knees most of the way and swing your arm structure forward and up, using the scapulae instead of the arm muscles. Direct the earth's force to your hands and fingers, and feel the spine being charged with the earth's force.

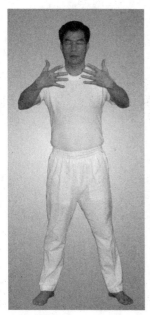
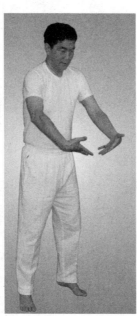
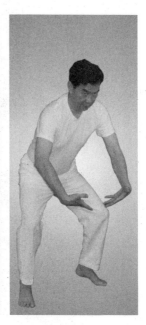

| Tendon Nei Kung sixth position | Tendon Nei Kung seventh position | Tendon Nei Kung eighth position |

TENDON NEI KUNG

🌀 **Partner Practice**

(Pages 63–76)

In these exercises, your partner leans on your wrists in each position. When you use the principles of Tendon Nei Kung to torque your tendons from the ankles upward, you gently bounce him away.

1. First position (hands at nose level and palms facing each other): Your partner leans inward on your wrists. Absorb and store his energy in your tendons, then torque your tendons—emphasizing the middle fingers—to bounce him away.

2. Second position (hands form the shape of a roof at eye level): Your partner leans in on your wrists. Absorb and store his energy in your tendons, then torque your tendons—emphasizing the pinkie fingers— to bounce him away.

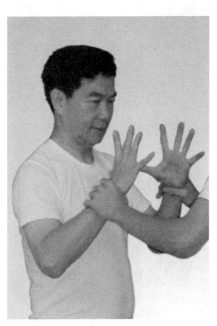
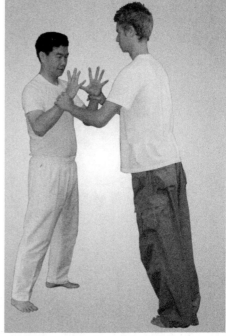

Second position with a partner

3. Third position (hands holding a "ball" at the abdomen): Partner leans in on the thumb side of your wrists. As you bounce him away, keep your elbows bent and extend your power from your shoulders.

4. Fourth position (hands palm down in front of abdomen): Partner leans in on the tops of your wrists. As you bounce him away, feel the chi rising up out of the backs of your hands.

5. Fifth position (hands at solar plexus in a "roof" shape): Partner leans in on the front of your wrists. As you bounce him away, focus on your pinkie tendons and use the spine's whiplike movement to generate force.

6. Sixth position (hands at shoulder level with palms facing you and elbows down): Your partner leans in on the spot where the thumb meets the wrist. As you bounce him away, emphasize the whiplike motion of the spine to generate force.

7. Seventh position (hands at waist height with palms up, forming a basket): Partner leans on the spot where the thumb joins the wrist. Before you bounce him away, be sure to lock your shoulder joints and use the spine's motion.

8. Eighth position (knees bent, hands forming a basket at knee level): Your partner will place his hands on your shoulders and lean in. Sink

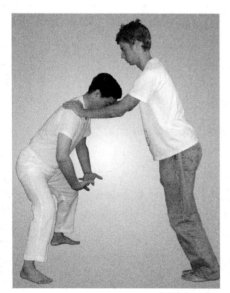 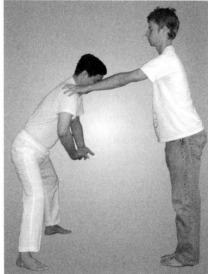

Eighth position with a partner

down and absorb his energy into your tendons. Torque your tendons and rise up a little bit to bounce him away. Feel the earth's force pulsing through your spine.

9. Closing movements: Shake out your body, then relax and smile to your tendons. Collect energy in the lower tan tien.

Wall Practice
(Pages 77–82)

For these exercises, stand about an arm's length away from the wall and fall against it slowly, then bounce yourself upright by torquing your tendons. A few of the positions from the previous exercise have been eliminated here, as they cannot be done against a wall.

1. First position (hands at nose level and palms facing each other): Lean into the wall on the backs of your hands and wrists. Expand onto your toes and torque your tendons to bounce yourself upright.

2. Second position (hands form the shape of a roof at eye level): Lean into the wall on the ulnar edge (pinkie side) of your hands. Absorb your momentum into your tendons, then expand onto your toes and torque your tendons to bounce yourself upright.

3. Fifth position (hands at solar plexus in a "roof" shape): Lean into the wall on the ulnar edge (pinkie side) of your hands. Absorb your momentum into your tendons, then expand onto your toes and torque your tendons to bounce yourself upright.

4. Sixth position (hands at shoulder level with palms facing you and elbows down): Lean into the wall on the backs of your hands. Engage your tendons to absorb and store your force, then torque to bounce yourself upright. Feel the whiplike motion of the spine.

5. Seventh position (hands at waist height with palms up, forming a basket): Lean into the wall on the backs of your wrists (at waist height). Engage your tendons to absorb and store your force, then torque to bounce yourself upright. Feel the whiplike motion of the spine.

6. Shake out your arms and legs, then collect energy at the navel.

TENDON NEI KUNG

✷ Mung Bean Hitting
(Pages 110–21)

For this exercise, strike your tendons with a cotton sock filled with 1 pound of mung beans. As you prepare each part of the body for hitting, swallow saliva down into your belly.

1. Arm: Extend your left arm and hit along the middle finger, pinkie, thumb, and back-of-the-hand lines. For each line, strike the elbow point 3 times, then hit along the line toward the hand. Return along the same route to the top of the neck, then back down to the elbow. Repeat the same sequence on the other arm.
2. Torso and leg: Stretch your left leg forward and hit along the big toe line (left shoulder, mid-torso, right leg), the little toe line (left armpit, left flank, right leg), the middle toe line (left shoulder, left-side organs, right leg), and the back-of-the-leg line (left side of spine, back of right leg). For each line, start hitting at the left shoulder and progress down the torso to the right leg and foot, then follow the same route back up to the neck. Repeat each line on the other side.

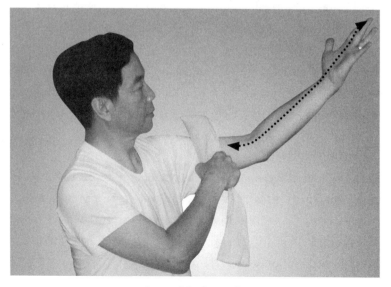

The middle finger line

FUSION OF THE EIGHT PSYCHIC CHANNELS

🌀 Formula 1: Opening the Great Bridge and Regulator Channels

(Pages 71–82)

1. Either sitting or standing, do the Inner Smile practice and the Fusion of the Five Elements and Cosmic Fusion practices. Take these purified energies into your lower tan tien and create a strong pearl. Bring it into your perineum.

2. Bring the pearl up through each of the three Thrusting Channels in succession. Inhale and draw the pearl up, then exhale and let all the toxins in the channel drain down into the earth. Return the pearl to the perineum.

3. Split the pearl into two pearls and draw them up the Left and Right Thrusting Channels to the GB 16 points on the top of the head. Place your middle fingers on these points and spiral them until they feel numb and tingling. Keeping the middle fingers in place, put your index fingers on GB 17 (1.5 inches behind GB 16) and your ring fingers on GB 15, and spiral them all until you feel the tingling sensation.

4. Move all three fingers to the GB 14 points. Pull the liquid chi from your crown to the forehead.

5. Place all three fingers on ST 2 and feel the energy drain down through your eyes to this point. Move your fingers to ST 4 and press slightly upward. Drain the infinite chi energy from your crown to this point.

🌸 The Yin Route

6. Keeping your fingers at ST 4, let the energy move to CV 23 (just under the chin). Press this point upward toward your tongue with either thumb. Press one thumb into your sternum, then press the index, middle, and ring fingers of your left hand into point CV 22. Let the energy drain down to this point.

7. Move the index, middle, and ring fingers of both hands to the ST 13

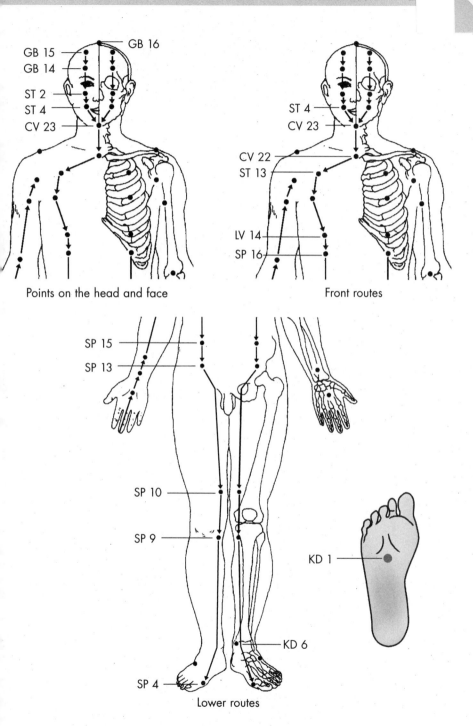

Points on the head and face

Front routes

Lower routes

Opening the Great Bridge and Regulator Channels

points. Massage them, then massage ST 16, just above the nipples. Move back to ST 13, then straight down to LV 14 (between the eighth and ninth ribs). Massage these points deeply, letting the energy sink into the bones, then move your fingers to just below the rib cage in line with the nipples—SP 16. Let the Golden Elixir flow into it.

8. Massage SP 15 (just below SP 16, level with the navel), SP 13 (below SP 15, at the top edge of the femur), SP 10 (above the medial side of the knee), and SP 9 (on the inner leg, below the knee). Let the elixir drain down to all of these points.

9. Massage KD 6 (one finger-width below the inner ankle bone), SP 4 (edge of the foot, two finger-widths below the ball joint of the big toe), and KD 1 (bottom of the foot). KD 1 is an antenna for earth energy, so open it wide while the elixir slowly flows in.

10. Clasp your hands and let the Golden Elixir flow from your crown to the soles of your feet.

🌸 The Yang Route

11. Place your fingers on GB 41 (between the fourth and fifth metatarsal bones). Let the energy flow up the outside of your leg in a straight line from UB 62 (one finger-width below the outer ankle bone) to GB 34 (just under the head of the fibula) to GB 31 (halfway to the hip joint).

12. Bring the energy onto your back through GB 29 (at the outer end of

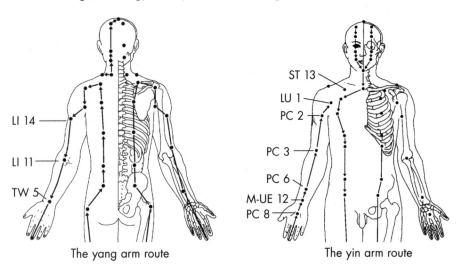

The yang arm route   The yin arm route

the crease when the hip is flexed) to UB 48. Move your right and left fingers to the back points: UB 47, UB 42, UB 38, then straight up the back to TW 15 at the top of your scapula. Massage the points SI 10 and SI 9 at the back of both armpits.

13. Clasp your hands. Let the energy move from your crown to the soles of your feet then up the back to SI 9. Let the energy tingle behind your eyes.

🌀 Linking the Yang and Yin Arm Routes

14. Put the three fingers of your right hand on the left arm's LI 14, then LI 11 (outer edge of the elbow crease), and TW 5 (two finger-widths behind the center of the back wrist crease). Let the Golden Elixir flow through these points.

15. Link the yang points to the yin points by bringing your right fingers to PC 8 (center of the palm) on the left palm. Move your fingers up along the yin side of the arm by touching M-UE 12, PC 6, PC 3, PC 2, and LU 1.

16. Rest and feel the elixir moving through the left arm, then repeat steps 14 and 15 on the right arm.

🌀 Upper Yang Routes

17. Place the fingers of both hands on the LU 1 points, then on LI 16. From there go to GB 21, M-HN 29, and GB 20 at the base of your skull.

18. Clasp your hands and let the energy dance slowly through the entire Great Bridge and Regulator Channels. Use your mind to link the two sides.

19. Collect energy at the navel and do Chi Self-Massage.

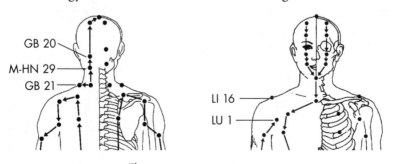

The upper yang route

FUSION OF THE EIGHT PSYCHIC CHANNELS
Energy Protection Formulas

⟳ Formula 2: Spinal Cord Cutting
(Pages 83–84)

This practice opens spinal blockages.

1. If starting fresh, do Fusion of the Five Elements practice to form a pearl, then circulate it several times through your Microcosmic Orbit.

2. Hold the pearl at the throat center, sending cosmic energy into it until the throat center starts to feel numb. Then inhale and exhale forcefully to project the pearl out from your throat.

3. Orbit the pearl over the top of your head to C7, then let it "cut through" your body at C7. Project the pearl out through the front of your body at this level, orbit it around your head to T1, then cut into your body again at T1.

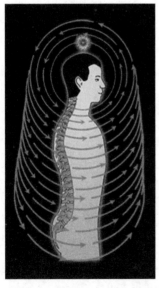
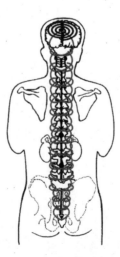
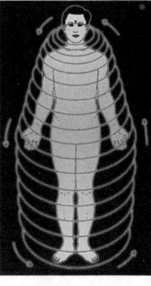

Spinal cord cutting	Spinal cord Microcosmic Orbit	Cutting from the third eye

4. Continue projecting the pearl out the front of your body and making progressively larger loops over your head, cutting into the next lowest vertebra each time. When the vertebrae are numb and tingling, continue orbiting and cutting through the sacrum and coccyx.

5. Finish by orbiting back upward in progressively smaller loops, until the pearl is back at the throat center.

Formula 3: Spinal Cord Microcosmic Orbit
(Pages 84–87)

1. Do Fusion of the Five Elements practice to form a pearl, then circulate it several times through your Microcosmic Orbit. Tighten your anus and let the pearl swim into your sacrum. Let the pearl slowly swim up inside your spine to the Jade Pillow point, then bring it into your brain. Wrap the pearl over your brain inside your skull, then slowly bring it down inside the front of your spinal column.

2. Let the pearl swim into the coccyx, then up the outside of the back of the spinal cord. Wrap it around your brain inside your skull, then down along the outside of the front of your spinal cord so that it encircles the whole spine.

3. Let the pearl swim into the coccyx, then up the outside of the back of your spinal cord deep into your brain. Spiral it around your skull, then down the inside of the spinal cord to the coccyx.

4. Repeat this spinal cord Microcosmic Orbit until the spinal cord is dripping with chi.

Formula 4: Cutting from the Third Eye
(Page 88)

1. Hold the pearl deep within your third eye, then project it out. Orbit it clockwise or counterclockwise to cut into and through your neck, then back up to the third eye.

2. Repeat this step again, orbiting in progressively larger loops to cut through each vertebra, driving the pearl deep into all the organs and glands.

3. Finish by cutting the pearl back into your third eye and letting the energy drain down past your throat and chest to spiral in the lower tan tien.

Formula 5: Drilling into the Head
(Page 89)

1. Move the pearl to your third eye and spiral it through your brain to the back of your head. Continue to drill horizontally from various points on the forehead and face to the back of the head, and from side to side. Drill deep into your eyes, nose, and ears. Be thorough.
2. Drill the pearl vertically from Pai Hui down to the chin. Drill vertically from points all over your crown. Feel the brain permeated with multi-orgasmic energy.

Formula 6: Cutting the Senses
(Pages 90–91)

Hold the pearl about a half-inch in front of your eyes, and spiral it deep under the skin in three figure-eight motions, as follows.

1. Spiral the pearl down to the bottom of the left eye, over and around the left ear, then up to the left eyebrow and back to the third eye.
2. From the third eye, spiral the pearl into the skin and down to the bottom of the right eye, over the top of the right ear, then down around the ear and up over the right eyebrow to the third eye.
3. From the third eye, spiral the pearl down the left side of your nose, then cross over to the right corner of your mouth. Circle around to the left corner of the mouth, then up the right side of the nose back to the third eye.

Formula 7: Butterfly Protection
(Pages 92–93)

1. Move pearl to the sternum and split it into two pearls. Beginning at ST 16 (just above the nipples), cut into the rib cage and spiral your pearls in outward and downward arcs like butterfly wings.

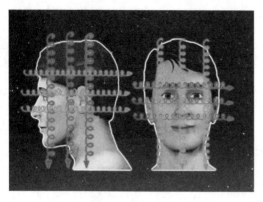

Drilling into the head

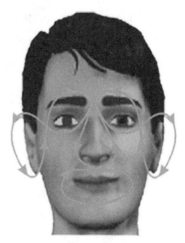

Cutting the senses

Drilling your head with energy

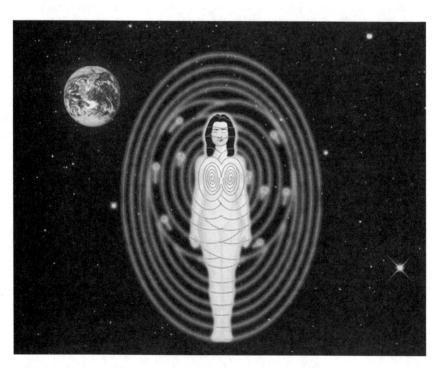

Butterfly Protection

2. Expand the spirals with each circuit until they eventually include your whole body, and your aura. Make 20 spirals, then collect energy at the navel and do Chi Self-Massage.

◉ Formula 8: Sealing the Aura
(Pages 93–96)

1. Spiral the pearl deep into your navel, then send it down the front of your right leg to the big toe. Cross over to the big toe of the left foot. Run energy up each toe of the left foot, then up the outer edge of the left leg and left side of the body to the armpit.
2. Trace energy up the inside of your left arm and hand, then the outside of the arm from fingers to shoulder. Now trace the energy over the crown to the right shoulder.
3. Move the pearl down the outside, then the inside of the right arm, then down the right side and right leg to the toes. Trace each toe, then bring a sheet of energy up the inside of the right leg, around the perineum, and down the inner left leg to the toes.
4. Bring the pearl up the front of the left leg to the pelvis, then cross the torso diagonally to reach the right collarbone. Trace down the inside of the right arm to the fingers, then up the outside of the arm and over the crown.
5. Move the energy from the left shoulder down the outside of the left arm, then up the inside of the left arm to the collarbone. Cross the torso diagonally downward to reach the right hip, then trace energy down the front of the right leg.
6. Draw the pearl up the back of the right leg and buttock to T11. Cross over T11 diagonally upward to reach the left scapula. Trace down the inside of the left arm, then up the outside to the shoulder and over the crown. Trace down the outside of the right arm, then up the inside to the right scapula. Move the energy diagonally downward to cross over T11 and run down the back of the right leg to the toes. Bring energy up the front of the left leg and collect it at the navel. Feel the aura around you and let your spirit implode with multi-orgasmic energy and compassion energy.

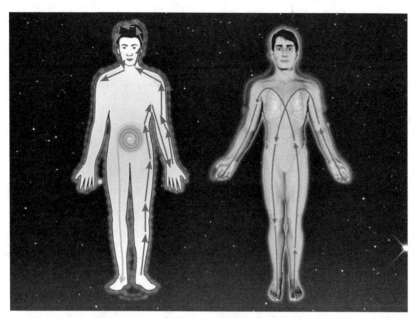

Sides   Front

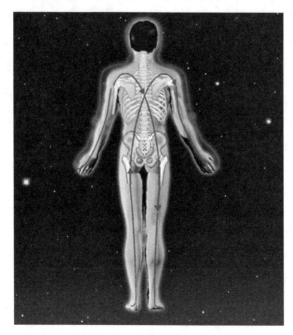

Back

Sealing the Aura

FUSION OF THE EIGHT PSYCHIC CHANNELS
Advanced Fusion Practice

🌀 Forming the Energy Body

(Pages 96–99)

1. Practice formulas 1–8 above, then bring the pearl to the perineum.

2. Inhale the life force in short sips—up to your navel, up to your heart, then up to your crown.

   Swallow your saliva upward and exhale forcefully to shoot the pearl out of the crown. Feel the pearl expanding with energy from the North Star, Big Dipper, and the cosmic particle force. Bring earth energy up from your feet and feel the pearl expand further.

3. Relax your senses as you form the energy body above your crown.

4. Run the Microcosmic Orbit in your physical body, then open your crown and copy the pathway of the Microcosmic Orbit into your energy body. Form another pearl in your physical body and shoot it into your energy body, circulating the pearl through both Microcosmic Orbits.

5. Move your Thrusting Channels into your energy body. Circulate energy through your Belt Channel, spiraling it up through your crown to encircle the energy body and the physical body, connecting all the channels and protecting them.

6. Practice formulas 1–8 in your energy body. Let your energy body travel carefully to absorb the energies of the North Star, Big Dipper, other stars, and the planets.

7. When you're ready, shrink your energy body into a pearl. Activate the cranial pump, look up at your crown, and activate the lead light. Draw the pearl down into the lead light and inhale it back into your crown.

8. Move the pearl through the Microcosmic Orbit to nourish your physical body with its energies, then bring it down to the cauldron. Spiral and condense all the energies in the cauldron. Finish with Chi Self-Massage.

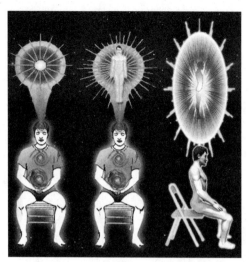

Extend the
Microcosmic
Orbit.

Extend the
Thrusting
Channels.

Extend the Belt
Channel.

Expanding the energy body

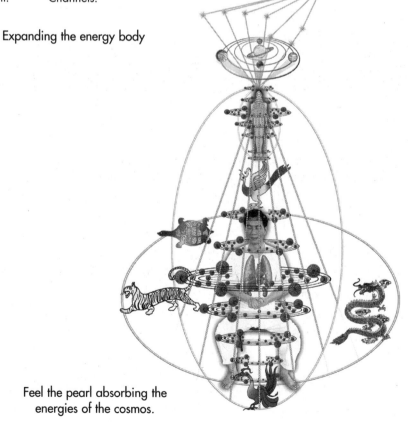

Feel the pearl absorbing the
energies of the cosmos.

Level Five

The fifth level of the Universal Healing Tao system corresponds to four Destiny Books editions of Universal Healing Tao books: *Taoist Astral Healing, Advanced Chi Nei Tsang, Golden Elixir Chi Kung,* and *Tai Chi Fa Jin.* These practices continue to refine the physical body's ability to channel the subtle energies of the earth and the cosmos.

TAOIST ASTRAL HEALING

Theory: Taoist Astral Healing is the second level of Cosmic Healing in the Universal Healing Tao Healing Arts. We call this practice "Cosmic Healing" because we ultimately learn to use the forces of nature, human will, and cosmic particles to transform negativity stored in the body. The Taoist recognizes that human beings have a limited capacity for chi. However, if we are able to connect with the sources of chi in the universe, we gain an infinite capacity for chi, and we constantly fill ourselves with the unlimited abundance of energy around us. This book specifically focuses on the teachings of Taoist astrology and explores how we can use this ancient wisdom about the energies of the cosmos in our spiritual and healing practice.

Concept: Taoist Astral Healing provides a step-by-step program for refining the ability to cultivate, circulate, and retain chi from the stars and planets. It offers advanced techniques for drawing down energies from the stars and planets in order to grow in awareness and to develop full soul potential. Harnessing these energies allows you to break through the cycles of attraction and addiction, promote longevity, and transform your physical and energy body into your light body in order to heal yourself and others as you discover your own divinity.

Purpose: The goal of our meditative practices is to tune in to the energy frequencies and awareness field of the planets and stars and integrate these into our physical body. As children of the universe, we are not only created by the divine intelligence and subtle substance of the cosmos, but if we allow it, we can also be co-creators of its evolutionary process.

ADVANCED CHI NEI TSANG

Theory: Advanced Chi Nei Tsang is the second level of the Chi Nei Tsang practices. It is based on the notion that every organ in the body has an intrinsic wind that flows and circulates in a healthy manner to support the maintenance of vitality. If there are blockages in the internal energy routes, the winds become renegade forces that throw the body further out of balance. Trapped wind is heavy, gray, and sick, like a damp room with no ventilation. Using Advanced Chi Nei Tsang is akin to opening the right windows to let the stagnant wind go out and to assist in reestablishing a healthy flow of vital energy.

Concept: Releasing the tension around the navel creates a space where the sick winds can gather in the way that water pools when you make a hole in the earth. It is an invitation for the winds to come to this area. Your work is to collect them there and then assist them by creating movement so they can leave the body, making space for healthy chi.

Purpose: Advanced Chi Nei Tsang will guide you deeper into the rib cage, abdomen, and navel center, teaching you how to use the elbow and knuckle techniques to release negative emotions, stress, tension, and sickness. These techniques are applied to the abdominal center where the universal, cosmic particle, and earth forces are combined and stored.

GOLDEN ELIXIR CHI KUNG

Theory: Thousands of years ago Taoists became aware of changes in the taste and consistency of saliva that accompanied meditative practices. They learned that combining saliva with the hormonal fluids and essences released during sexual activities forms a powerful elixir. Taoists believe that this Golden Elixir is not only a physical healing agent but also is a major transformative agent in preparing for higher spiritual (energy) work.

Concept: Golden Elixir Chi Kung contains twelve postures that develop and utilize the healing power of saliva. Ten of these involve gathering energy and forces through the body's hair, which acts as a negative energy filter and can also be used to store surplus positive energy. These practices will help you develop self-healing abilities that revitalize organs and promote longevity and spiritual vitality.

Purpose: The practices of Golden Elixir Chi Kung use the energies of the saliva, hormonal fluids, and chi to create the potent Golden Elixir for health, healing, and spiritual transformation.

TAI CHI FA JIN

Theory: Tai Chi Fa Jin is the Tai Chi Chi Kung Discharge Form of the Universal Healing Tao system. Discharge power is the ability of the practitioner to issue force or power without evident effort. It involves the cultivation of power deep within and a calculated discharge of that power in a highly focused and carefully executed form.

Concept: The Tai Chi Chi Kung Discharge Form is a Yang style form with thirteen movements (eight gates and five positions) in four directions, beginning in the north and moving counterclockwise 360 degrees then clockwise 360 degrees. The steps required to accomplish Fa Jin will be explained through the lens of practices taught within the Universal Healing Tao system, including Iron Shirt structure, the transfer of power from the tan tien and turning of the waist as taught in the basic form of

Tai Chi Chi Kung and Tan Tien Chi Kung, and the coupling of yin and yang as taught in the Fusion practices and Kan and Li meditations.

Purpose: Fa Jin is the transformation of an opponent's yang and tension energy, which is neutralized deep in the earth and the lower tan tien, and combined with yin energy. From this coupling there is an explosion of jin, which is then discharged back to the opponent. By doing your daily Fa Jin practice, you imprint the form into your energy body, so that you will take the form and its movements with you to the next level of existence when you leave your physical body.

TAOIST ASTRAL HEALING

◎ Meditation 1: Earth-Sun-Moon Triangle
(Pages 167–71)

Before any Taoist Astral Healing practice, it is important to "warm up" your being with several basic exercises from Cosmic Chi Kung, Tai Chi, Tao Yin, etc.

1. Open the three tan tiens to the six directions, then practice the Inner Smile and Microcosmic Orbit.

2. Connect to Mother Earth force: exhale deeply into the earth and inhale cool blue energy into your palms, soles, and perineum. Store this energy in your lower tan tien.

3. Bring your attention to your sacrum and picture a bright full silver-white moon behind you, shining on your sacrum. Breathe moonlight through the sacrum into your sexual center, where it mixes with blue sexual energy. Pull up on your anus, perineum and sexual organs, and gently squeeze the muscles around the prostate/uterus and ovaries. Practice this for 5–10 minutes.

4. Bring your attention to your mid-eyebrow point and picture a bright

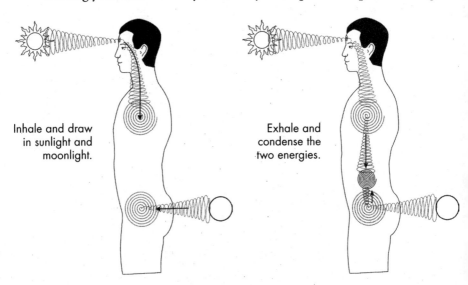

Inhale and draw in sunlight and moonlight.

Exhale and condense the two energies.

Connecting the sun and moon energy in the body

golden sun in front of you. Absorb the tingling light particles into your third eye and pituitary gland. Breathe in the light and guide it from the third eye and pituitary gland down to the heart.

5. Make the heart's sound (haw-w-w-w-w-w) to clean and balance the heart's energy. Feel love, peace, patience, and respect as the sun shines into your heart. Blend the golden yellow color of sunlight with the bright red color of love and compassion in your heart center (behind the sternum, right between your nipples). Gather more sunlight until you feel the "blooming of compassion."

6. Inhale silver white moonlight into the sacrum and sexual center and golden yellow sunlight into the third eye and heart center at the same time. Exhale and condense these two energies behind your navel, bringing heart energy down through the aorta and sexual energy up through the vena cava. Continue for 10–15 minutes until the lower tan tien and the body are vibrating with orgasmic energy.

7. Move this energy into the perineum and circulate it in the Microcosmic Orbit 9–18 times. Feel your perineum connect to the earth, your sacrum connect to the moon, your crown connect to the North Star and Big Dipper, and your third eye connect to the sun.

8. Gather energy in your lower tan tien and rest. Finish with Chi Self-Massage.

Meditation 2: Strengthening the Organs and Balancing the Emotions
(Pages 171–75)

1. Open the three tan tiens to the six directions, then practice the Inner Smile and Microcosmic Orbit.

2. Make a firm chi ball in the lower tan tien and connect to the earth force. Touch your cranial bones very lightly—with a "butterfly touch"—and feel your craniosacral rhythm. Expand your awareness of this rhythm 5–50 centimeters away from your physical body.

3. Place your nondominant hand on your spleen/pancreas and fill these organs with the yellow light of openness and trust. Form a beak with

your dominant hand and place it softly on your crown to connect with the sphenoid bone.

4. Let chi move between your hands and between the spleen/pancreas and sphenoid bone. When you feel the connection, hold your hands in front of your tan tien, expand your cranial structure, and look up with your eyes through your crown. Visualize Saturn, and let its bright yellow light shine down into your crown, directly into your sphenoid bone, spleen, and pancreas, charging them with energy.

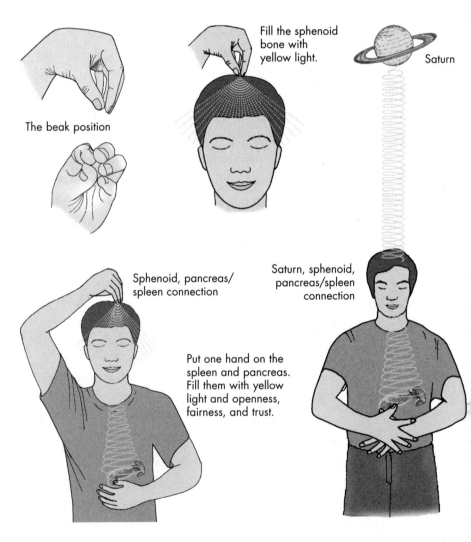

Fill the sphenoid bone with yellow light.

Saturn

The beak position

Sphenoid, pancreas/ spleen connection

Saturn, sphenoid, pancreas/spleen connection

Put one hand on the spleen and pancreas. Fill them with yellow light and openness, fairness, and trust.

Spleen/pancreas, sphenoid bone, and Saturn

5. Place your nondominant hand on your lungs and your flat dominant hand lightly on your left parietal bone. Fill them with the white light of courage and righteousness. Repeat step 4 to connect your lungs and left parietal bone, and fill them with the white light of Venus.

6. Place one hand on your liver and the other (flat hand) on your right parietal bone. Fill them with the green light of kindness. Repeat step 4 to connect your liver and right parietal bone to Jupiter, charging them with its clear green energy.

7. Place one hand on your heart and the other on your frontal bone. Fill them with the red light of love, peace, and respect. Repeat step 4 to connect your heart and frontal bone to Mars, and to fill them with its warm red energy.

8. Place one hand on the Door of Life point and the other on the occipital bone. Fill them with the blue light of gentleness. Repeat step 4 to connect your kidneys and occipital bone to Mercury, charging them with its deep blue energy.

9. Visualize all five planets above your crown, and let their light shine into the cranial entrances, deeply connecting to the organs. Bring all these energies together in the lower tan tien and condense them into a chi ball. Circulate the chi ball in the Microcosmic Orbit 9–18 times.

10. Gather energy in the lower tan tien and finish with Chi Self-Massage.

Meditation 3: Strengthening Energy Fields
(Pages 176–79)

1. Repeat meditation 2 from the previous pages. This time, connect the organs, cranial bones, and planets to the element they are associated with, as follows: spleen/earth; lungs/metal; liver/wood; heart/fire; kidneys/water. Spend time connecting to these elemental forces, then mix the elemental and planetary energies in the organs.

2. Let the energy, color, and virtue of each organ expand into its related body system as follows, then let it expand out into your aural field:

3. Spleen/sphenoid bone/Saturn/earth element/muscular or lymphatic system.

4. Lungs/left parietal/Venus/metal element/respiratory system.

5. Liver/right parietal/Jupiter/wood element/tendon and ligament system.

6. Heart/frontal bone/Mars/fire element/circulatory system.

7. Kidneys/occipital bone/Mercury/water element/bone structure and hormonal system.

8. Feel the strong, multicolored energy filling and surrounding your whole body, then add the sun and moon energy: Sun/fire element/pericardium/third eye/lymph and immune system; Moon/water element/sexual organs/sacrum/hormonal system.

9. Envision all the planets above and round you, and let their energies move freely through your body. Condense these energies into a chi ball in your lower tan tien, and circulate it in the Microcosmic Orbit. Gather again in the lower tan tien and rest, ending with Chi Self-Massage.

Meditation 4: Connecting to the Stellar and Galactic Forces

(Pages 179–85)

1. Open the three tan tiens to the six directions, then practice the Inner Smile and Microcosmic Orbit.

2. Make a firm, condensed chi ball in the lower tan tien and connect to the earth force.

3. Connect the six galaxies in six directions with golden light.

4. Connect with the North Star and five palaces, expanding your awareness beyond the Milky Way and into the galaxy around the North Star.

5. Circulate the energy in the Microcosmic Orbit, and then collect energy at the navel and do Chi Self-Massage.

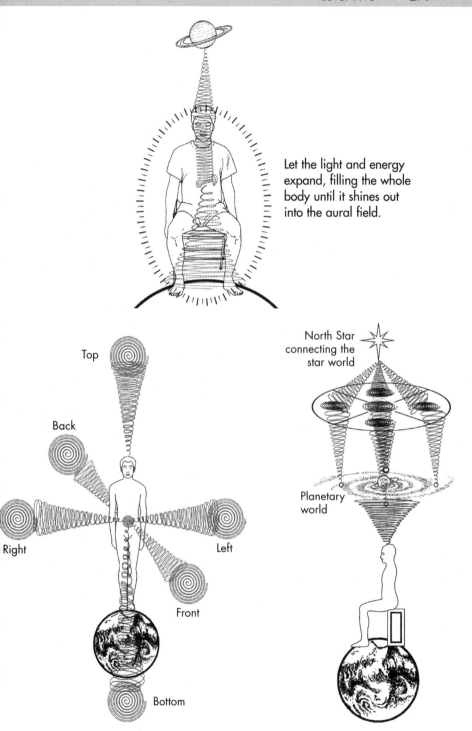

Let the light and energy expand, filling the whole body until it shines out into the aural field.

North Star connecting the star world

Top

Back

Right

Left

Front

Planetary world

Bottom

Galaxy connection with the five palaces in the six directions

Meditation 5: Balancing the Planetary and Stellar Influences

(Pages 185–88)

Before you begin this practice, determine which elemental force is the strongest in your being and which the weakest.

1. Open the three tan tiens to the six directions, then practice the Inner Smile and Microcosmic Orbit.
2. Condense a firm chi ball in the lower tan tien and connect with the Mother Earth force.
3. Connect the organs, cranial bones, planets, galaxies, and elemental forces as in the above meditations.

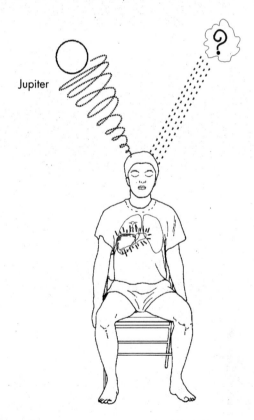

Jupiter

Balancing the energy: Jupiter influence reflects strong Liver Chi, while Venus influence weakens Lung Chi.

4. Identify your strongest element (Jupiter/liver in this example), and ฀฀฀ your body with its color—in this case, green.

5. Now change the color in your body and auric field to the color of your weakest system—in this example white/Venus/lungs. Place both hands over the lungs and draw the white color in. Place one hand on your left parietal bone and feel its connection to the lungs.

6. When you feel the connection, place your hands in front of your navel and turn your eyes to the left, upward, and inward—looking through the parietal bone and out through the skull in the direction of Venus and the white galaxy. Visualize a clear white ball above you and let its energy shine directly into your body.

7. Repeat this transition from strongest to weakest element several times until their energies feel more balanced. If it doesn't work, let the color of the strongest system (green, in this case) project through the weakest system (through the left parietal bone/Venus/white galaxy, in this example) until you feel the color of the weak system clearly. Then let this color fill your whole body—especially the respiratory system—and aura.

8. Condense a chi ball in the lower tan tien and circulate it in the Microcosmic Orbit. Gather it again in the lower tan tien and rest, then finish with Chi Self-Massage.

Meditation 6: Balancing Yin/Yang Extremes in the Star World

(Pages 188–90)

Take time to master the previous five meditations before attempting this one, as it can be harmful to a practitioner who is not well prepared.

1. Start with the warm-ups and practices recommended for the previous meditations, making sure to establish a good grounding.

2. Expand your awareness to the star world. Connect with the North Star and the Big Dipper, letting their light fill your upper tan tien. Visualize two points on either side of the North Star: one an extreme light/yang point (quasar) and the other an extreme dark/yin point (black hole).

3. Visualize these two points circling around the North Star faster and faster. Continue letting them circle around as you move your awareness into and through the North Star.

4. At a certain point, these points will be orbiting so fast that the boundaries between yin and yang will start to fall away and you will feel a lifting sensation. Let the process continue until yin and yang melt together, giving rise to pure yang energy.

5. Return to the place of Wu Chi—nothingness—and rest, letting the practice do its work.

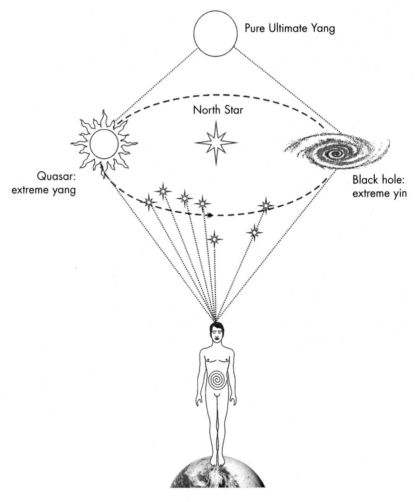

Pure Ultimate Yang

North Star

Quasar:
extreme yang

Black hole:
extreme yin

Balancing yin and yang

⟳ Meditation 7: Yin Stage Awareness
(Pages 191–94)

1. Warm up, then open the three tan tiens to the six directions and do the Inner Smile practice and Microcosmic Orbit.
2. Condense a firm chi ball in the lower tan tien and connect to Mother Earth energy.
3. Bring your attention to your cranial rhythm and expand it into your aural field. (If you are meditating with a group, connect to the energy fields of those in the group at this time.)
4. Relax and be receptive. Observe the energies that are influencing you from moment to moment: the specific nature entities, planets, individual stars, elemental forces, galaxies, pulsars, quasars, black holes, etc.
5. At the end of the meditation, draw the energy back into your own individual field. Condense a chi ball in your lower tan tien and circulate it in your Microcosmic Orbit. Gather it again in your lower tan tien and rest. Finish with Chi Self-Massage.

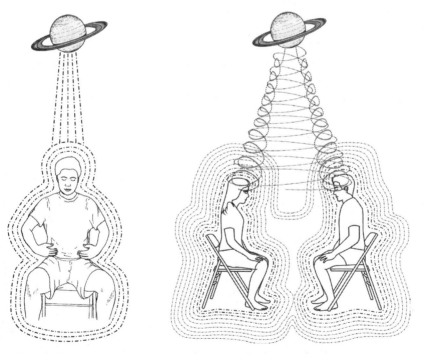

Individual and two-person awareness meditation with Saturn influence

ADVANCED CHI NEI TSANG

Opening the Wind Gates at the Navel
(Pages 40–49)

1. Upper left quadrant: Press your elbow down on the navel and move it toward your student's left (W/270°). Repeat this movement from the center outward, moving in ten-degree increments up toward the S/180° point, then returning to W/270° in the same way.

2. Lower left quadrant: Release the pressure, then press down and out from 270° to 360°/N in ten-degree increments, then back to 270°.

3. Have the student breathe in deeply to push your elbow out. Flush the winds down the legs and out through the toes.

4. Lower right quadrant: Press with your elbow toward the student's right—E/90°. Repeat the steps above on the lower right quadrant from 90° toward 0° and from 0° toward 90°.

5. Repeat for the upper right quadrant—from 90° toward 180°. Flush and vent 15–20 times.

Making Space in the Pakua
If there's too much wind when pressing down, stop, flush, and vent.

6. Press both hands or thumbs on the northern gate at the bottom of the pakua (0/360°: bladder/genitals). Repeat at the southern gate (top of pakua, heart, 180°); the eastern gate (right side of the pakua, right kidney, 90°); the western gate (left side, left kidney, 270°); the southwestern gate (upper left, stomach/spleen, 225°); the northeastern gate (lower right, intestines, 45°); the southeastern gate (upper right, liver/gallbladder, 135°); and the northwestern gate (lower left, intestines, 315°). Flush and vent 15–20 times.

7. Have your student press her fingers on her navel and feel a fire in her lower tan tien burning out the sick winds.

8. Close session with Monkey Dancing: Have student lie on her back and raise her arms and legs up. Shake them enthusiastically while laughing and breathing deeply into abdomen.

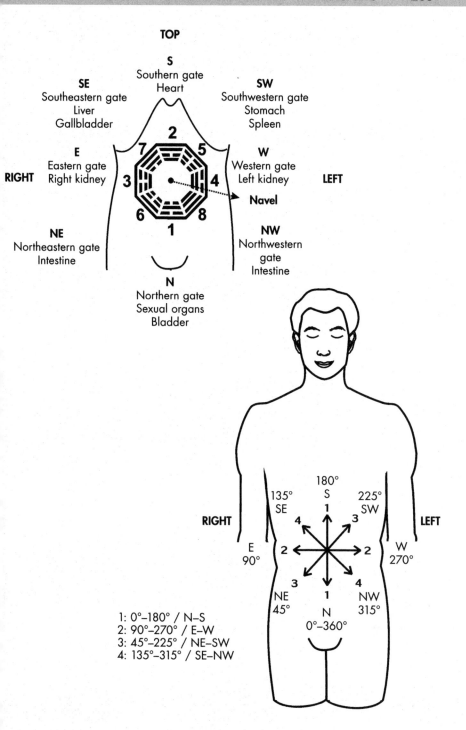

Sequence for releasing the wind gates

ADVANCED CHI NEI TSANG
Working on the Winds

⟳ The First Wind: Liver, Pericardium, and Heart
(Pages 52–57)

Press the points with your elbow. Flush out wind after each point.

1. Press point 35 (above the navel, left and right) and point 32 (below the navel, left and right).
2. Press point 37 (above the navel, left and right) and point 30 (below the sternum).
3. Release wind by loosening under the ribs and massaging the liver. Have student make the liver's sound (sh-h-h-h-h-h).

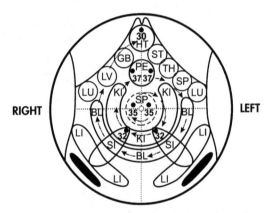

Navel points for the first and second winds

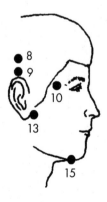
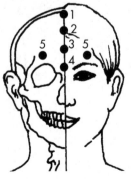
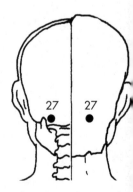

Points on the head

4. Press your knuckles gently into points 22 and 23 on the left side of the ribcage (above the nipple, or between fourth and fifth ribs); spiral counterclockwise. Have student make the heart's sound (haw-w-w-w-w-w) and the triple warmer's sound (hee-e-e-e-e-e).

5. Flush winds from heart area by spiraling your hand above the heart and down along the left arm.

6. Repeat steps 4 and 5 on the right side.

7. Release the sternum and heart area with your knuckle, working around the breasts on women. Flush down along the left arm.

8. Press point 53 (above the knee). Find it by laying your hand directly over the student's knee. Extend your thumb to inside of the student's leg, grab the thigh muscle, and press with your thumb. Flush wind down, then repeat this step on the other leg.

The Second Wind: Tongue, Eyes, and Head
(Pages 58–65)

1. Massage the soft area under the chin and press point 15 (under chin).

2. Massage jawbone back/forward/under with thumbs. Have student tighten and loosen the jaw by clenching his teeth and then opening his mouth repeatedly while you massage both sides.

3. Press your knuckle on point 13 (below the earlobe, at jaw edge). Work on both sides while student makes the liver's sound subvocally (sh-h-h-h-h-h).

4. Place your knuckle at a 90-degree angle on point 2 (center point above hairline); massage in a spiral.

5. Press point 3 (mid-forehead), point 4 (mid-eyebrow), and point 5 (above eyebrows). Massage the upper eye socket with your thumb.

6. Turn the student's head and spiral your knuckle on point 10 (outer edge of each eye). Do both sides together. Spiral your knuckle on points 8 and 9 (on the centerline above each ear), massaging both sides together.

7. Spiral knuckle on point 27 (Wind Pond, above the base of the skull, on both sides of the centerline) and make a curlicue to release stagnant chi. Gather winds with swirling hands into earth.

✿ The Third Wind: Kidneys

(Pages 66–72)

Use your elbow on student's navel points to loosen the small intestine.

1. Alternate inhaling into the heart and exhaling with the heart's sound (haw-w-w-w-w-w), with inhaling into the kidneys and exhaling with the kidneys' sound (choo-oo-oo-oo).

2. Press points 35 (just above navel) and 33 (just below navel) on the left, then on the right.

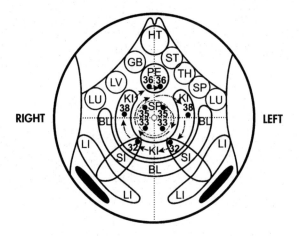

Navel points for the third wind

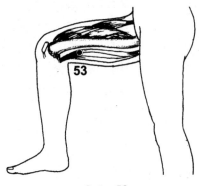

Point 53

3. Press point 38 (beside navel) on the left side, then point 32 (below navel, away from centerline) on the left side. Then press point 32 and 38 on the right.

4. Press point 36 (above navel, away from centerline) first on the right side then on the left. Flush out through knee point 53 (inner thigh muscle).

5. Press knuckle on point 8 (above ear) while supporting head with your other hand. Work on both sides.

6. Press point 53 (inner thigh). Flush wind down and repeat on the other side.

☯ The Fourth Wind: Vena Cava, Aorta, and Lumbar Plexus

(Pages 73–79)

1. Press point 32 (below navel) on the left then the right.

2. Press points 41 (lower tip of hip bone) and point 40 (on hip bone) on the right side, then 40 and 41 on the left side.

3. Press point 48 (upper leg) on the left then the right. Use tip of finger for this point.

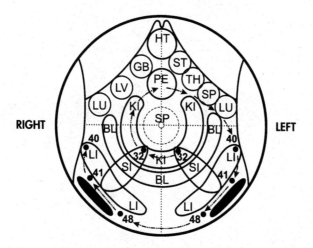

Navel points for the fourth wind

The following points need to be done on one side only—usually the left.

4. With student lying on her back, press point 21 (below collarbone).

5. With student sitting up, press points 20 (above collarbone), 75 (outer edge of shoulder), and 25 (armpit, with student's arm raised).

6. Massage the Heart meridian (inside of the left arm), down to the pinkie finger, pressing point 77 (inner elbow) along the way. Pinch the corners of the pinkie nail. Flush winds down the left arm.

7. Press your thumbs on point 69 or 54 (behind kneecap) and point 55 (above outer shin, below knee).

8. Press your thumbs on point 66 (inside of foot, below ankle). Flush wind down legs.

9. Press elbow on point 45 (between sacrum and hip). Flush wind down legs.

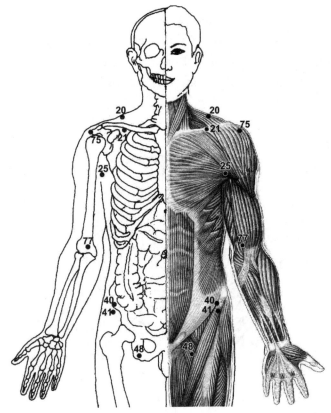

Points on the chest and shoulders

☯ The Fifth Wind: Abdomen

(Pages 80–83)

Use your elbow to press the navel points. Remember to flush wind out after each point.

1. Press point 35 on the left side (just above the navel), then point 33 on the left side (just below the navel). The press point 33 and 35 on the right side.
2. Press point 36 (above point 35) first on the right, then on the left.

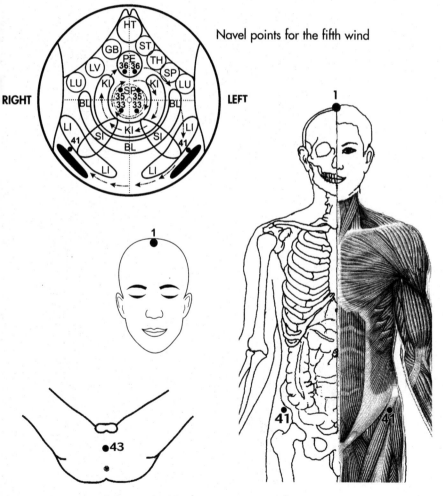

Navel points for the fifth wind

Points on inguinal area, crown, and perineum

3. Press point 41 on the left side, then the right (on the lower tip of the hip bone).

4. Spiral and hold your knuckle on point 1 (Crown point) as student connects with perineum and presses point 43 (perineum). Flush/vent from head down the arms and out through the legs.

5. Spiral with thumbs or elbows on point 57 (inner calf below knee), then use thumbs on point 66 (below inner ankle).

⊙ The Sixth Wind: Muscle Cramps

(Pages 84–88)

The navel points for the sixth wind are the same as those for the fifth wind.

1. Press point 35 on the left side (just above the navel), then point 33 on the left side (just below the navel). Then press points 33 and 35 on the right side.

2. Press point 36 (above point 35) first on the right, then on the left.

3. Press thumb on point 15 (under the chin), then press knuckle into point 13 (edge of jaw, below earlobe).

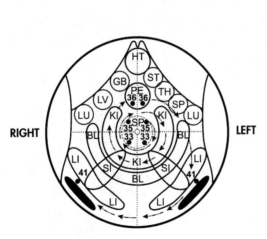

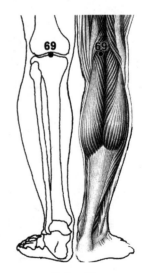

Navel points for the sixth wind

Point 69

4. Stretch student's calves and Achilles tendons by pushing the feet toward the navel and rotating them in a circle.

5. With student laying on stomach, press point 69 (behind knees, between the two muscles). Flush wind down the legs.

6. Slapping technique: With an open palm, slap the back of the leg, arm, wrist, or ankle. Strike sharply to create a stinging sensation. Do not work on varicose veins. Flush the wind down.

7. Close session with Monkey Dancing: Have student lie on his back and raise his arms and legs up. Shake them enthusiastically while laughing and breathing deeply into the abdomen.

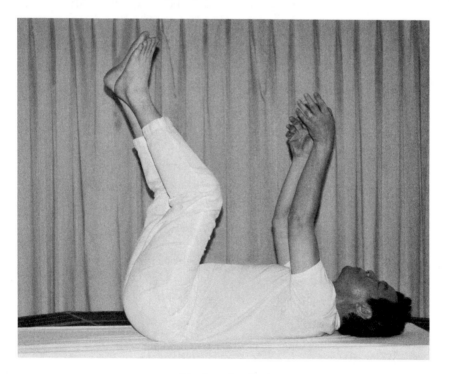

Monkey dancing

⊙ The Seventh Wind: Heart

(Pages 89–92)

1. Press point 35 (above navel) on the left side and point 33 (below navel) also on the left side. Then press points 33 and 35 on the right.
2. Press point 38 (to the side of the navel) on the left and the right, then point 36 (above navel) on the right and left.
3. Support your student's face with one hand and press your knuckle on point 13 (below ear) with the other hand.
4. Press point 74 (Bubbling Spring, on the sole of the foot) while your student pulls her toes toward her navel. Have her bring kidney energy up from the feet along the insides of her legs to the perineum, then into the lower abdomen, around the kidneys, and rising to the heart.
5. As you flush wind out through the feet, ask your student to make the heart's sound (haw-w-w-w-w-w) while drawing heat from the heart down to the kidneys, lower back, legs, and out through the toes to the earth. Encourage student to swallow saliva and belch frequently.

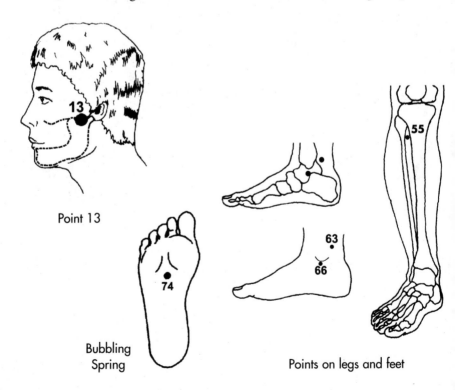

Point 13

Bubbling
Spring

Points on legs and feet

⟳ The Eighth Wind: Chest
(Pages 92–95)

1. Press point 35 on the left (just above navel) and point 33 (just below navel) also on the left. Then press points 33 and 35 on the right.
2. Press point 38 (beside navel) on the left and point 32 (below navel, away from centerline) also on the left. Then press points 32 and 38 on the right.
3. Press point 37 (above navel) on the right side, then the left. Press point 30 (just below the sternum). Be careful not to press on the tip of the sternum, which is very delicate.
4. Massage chest area using the heel of the palm. Spiral and shake your palm heel, then press your knuckle on and between the ribs. Encourage student to breathe into the pain.
5. Massage sternum with knuckle, gently on the sternum's tip. Flush wind down through the arms.

⟳ The Ninth Wind: Legs and Feet
(Pages 95–99)

1. Press point 35 (just above navel) on the left and point 33 (just below navel) also on the left. Then press points 33 and 35 on the right.
2. Press point 36 (above the navel) on the right side, then on the left.
3. Press knuckle into point 22 (just above nipples) on both sides. On women, this point can be found approximately between the fourth and fifth ribs. Flush wind down the arms.
4. Press point 40 on the left side (just above hip bone) and point 41 also on the left side (lower tip of hip bone).
5. Press point 49 on the left side (inside lower pelvic bone), on the left side.
6. Then press points 49, 41, and 40 on the right side. Flush winds down the legs.
7. On the left foot press points 63 (behind inner ankle bone) and 66 (below inner ankle bone). Then press point 55 on the left (front of leg below the knee) and flush the wind down the leg.
8. Press points 63, 66, and 55 on the right leg, and flush the wind down the leg.

☼ The Tenth Wind: Pain, Numbness, and Heat

(Pages 99–103)

While working on the navel points below, rest a finger on point 19 in the notch of the sternum.

1. Press point 35 (just above navel) on the left side, then the right. Then press point 36 (above point 35) on the right side, then the left. Flush winds down the arms.
2. With your knuckle, thumb, or finger, press point 19 (notch in upper sternum) and point 18 on both sides (above clavicle, near point 19).
3. Massage point 17 on both sides (on throat, below the notch on the vocal cords).
4. With your elbow, press point 20 (brachial plexus) while student turns his head from side to side. Work on both sides, then press your thumb on point 25 (in the armpit). Flush wind down the arms.
5. On either foot, press points 67 (inside of foot, below and forward from ankle bone) and 66 (inside of foot below anklebone).
6. Press point 74 (Bubbling Spring, on the sole of the foot) while supporting student's foot.
7. Press points 67, 66, and 74 on the other foot. Flush winds out.

☼ The Eleventh Wind: Nerves and Back

(Pages 103–6)

1. Press point 35 on the left (just above the navel) and point 33 on the left (just below the navel). Then press points 33 and 35 on the right.
2. Press point 38 on the left (beside navel) and point 32 on the left (below the navel, away from the centerline). Then press points 32 and 38 on the right. Press point 37 (above navel) on the right side, then the left.
3. Press point 30 (just below sternum). Do not press on the delicate tip of the sternum.
4. Massage below the navel with your fingers, then have student place

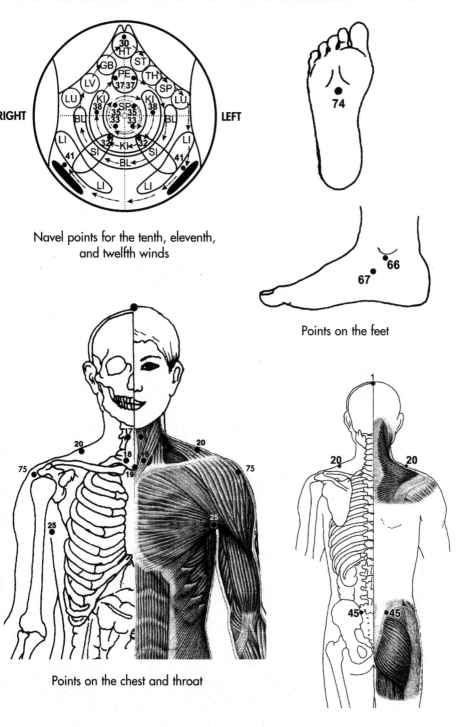

Navel points for the tenth, eleventh, and twelfth winds

Points on the feet

Points on the chest and throat

Points on the back

his palms over navel area while imagining a fire or burning sun baking his abdomen.

5. Massage point 75 (in deltoid muscle on outer shoulder) on both sides and point 20 (on shoulders at the base of the neck) on both sides. Flush winds out through the arms.

6. Press your elbow on point 45 (between sacrum and hip bone). Shake your arm and slightly push the hip bone down toward buttocks. Flush wind down through legs and feet.

☉ The Twelfth Wind: Heat and Cold
(Pages 107–9)

1. Press point 35 on the left (just above the navel) and point 33 on the left (just below the navel). Then press points 33 and 35 on the right.

2. Press point 38 on the left (beside navel) and point 32 on the left (below the navel, away from the centerline). Then press points 32 and 38 on the right.

3. Press point 37 (above navel) on the right side, then the left.

4. Press point 30 (just below sternum). Do not press on the delicate tip of the sternum.

5. Press point 41 (on the lower tip of the hip bone) on the left side, then the right.

6. Massage the sternum with your knuckle, also working on and between the ribs. Work around women's breasts. Have student make the heart's sound (haw-w-w-w-w-w) and release any excess heat or cold through the feet.

7. Flush wind down from left side of chest through the left arm and from right side of chest through right arm.

8. While supporting student's foot with one hand, press point 74 (on the sole of the foot) with your elbow. Flush the wind out.

ADVANCED CHI NEI TSANG
Applications for Specific Ailments

✷ Heart Attacks/The Life and Death Point
(Pages 110–12)

During an acute heart attack, the point between T4 and T6 on the left will be protruding noticeably and should be massaged with your elbow until the protrusion recedes.

1. Stand behind a sitting person or lay him comfortably face down.
2. Locate the protruding/pulsing point between T4 and T6 on the left side, between the scapula and the spine. Press your knuckle or elbow into it until it recedes.
3. Spiral your hand above this point to direct the wind down the person's left arm and hand; move it out of the body and into the ground.
4. After the emergency technique, massage the same point on the right side. Then massage the liver, gallbladder, duodenum, and both intestines, paying special attention to the ileocecal valve.

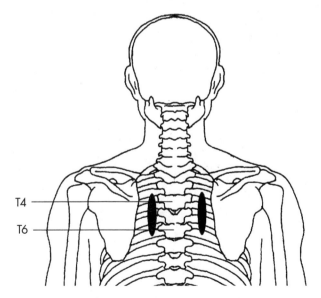

The Life and Death point on the left and the
corresponding point on the right

5. Remove wind from the liver (see techniques for the First Wind on page 286. Move the winds down the legs and feet, then out of the body and into the earth.

☯ Heart/Kidney/Breast Blockages
(Pages 113–14)

1. Open the Life and Death point with your knuckle.
2. Spiral your hand over the area to gather the stagnant chi, then sweep it down the arm and out through the hand.
3. Repeat steps 1 and 2 on the other side, then flush the wind down the arms.
4. Massage the area around the top and sides of the pubic bone, then flush the wind down the legs. Have student repeat this massage every day at home.

☯ Releasing Anger in the Jaw and Liver
(Page 115)

1. Use your knuckle to massage point 24 on the right side (on the lowest ribs, over the liver).
2. Hold the head steady, cup your fingers under the opposite side of the jaw, and use your thumb to release point 13 (under the chin). Repeat on opposite side of the jaw.

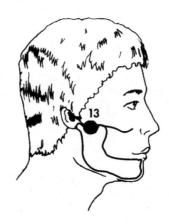

Point 13

Arthritis

Do not perform this massage on varicose veins.

1. Legs: Kneel beside a standing student and hold the front of the knee in one hand. With the other palm, swiftly slap the back of the knee 9–36 times. Repeat on other leg.
2. Arms: Grip the student's elbow, and slap the inside of the arm at the elbow crease 18 times. Repeat on the other arm.

Hiatal Hernia

(Pages 118–20)

1. Open the wind gates, the navel, and the pakua.
2. Massage the abdomen, releasing knots and tangles in the stomach and intestines. Focus on the upper left corner, just below the stomach.
3. Spiral and release the wind down the arms and legs.
4. Have student make the spleen's, heart's, lung's, and liver's sounds.

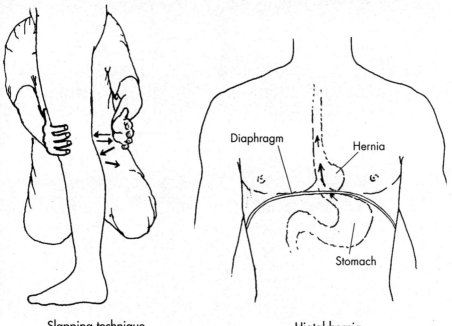

Slapping technique   Hiatal hernia

GOLDEN ELIXIR CHI KUNG

⊙ Dragon Gazes at the Pearl

(Pages 67–77)

1. Standing with your feet shoulder-width apart, make "dragon eyes" with your thumbs and index fingers and look through them. Close your eyes and practice "reverse breathing" by pulling in the lower abdomen as you inhale and expanding it as you exhale, keeping the chest relaxed.

2. Focus your awareness on the hair of your head (or on the follicles of the scalp if you are bald). Lightly touch your scalp and hair, and focus until you can feel the energy coming in through your hair as you inhale.

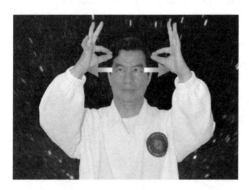

Dragon eyes

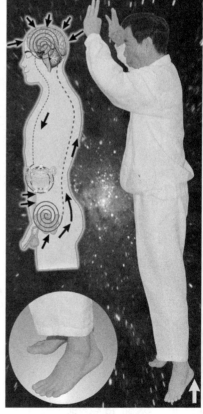

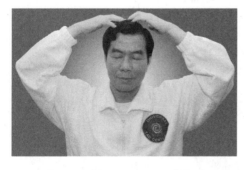

Touching and being aware of the hair

Rise up onto toes.

3. Become aware of your heart and tongue. As you inhale, feel each hair as an antenna, drawing Universal Chi toward you. As you exhale, feel the energy filtering through your hair, which transforms it from raw Universal Chi into energy that is useful for the organs and the body. Feel as if your hair is breathing.

4. Focus on the hair in your armpits (or the follicles, if you shave your armpits) and feel the connection between the spleen and the mouth. Inhale and gently pull your eyes in and your anus and perineum upward. At the same time, draw energy in through the armpit hair. As you exhale, relax your eyes and anus. Continue breathing through the armpit hair for about 30 seconds, then direct the energy from your armpits up your shoulders and into your mouth.

5. Draw energy into your mouth by sucking gently on your tongue and drawing in your cheeks as you move your lower jaw slowly forward and backward. Draw in nature and Universal Chi.

6. Place your hands in the "dragon-eyes" position from step 1, then inhale and rise up onto your toes as you gently pull the middle part of the anus up toward your head.

7. Draw all your energy into your mouth to join the energy from your head hair and armpit hair. Inhale and suck your eyes into your sockets, draw your tongue toward your throat, draw the ears in toward the ear canals, draw all your senses into the mouth, and suck in your cheeks. Hold your breath and pull in tighter.

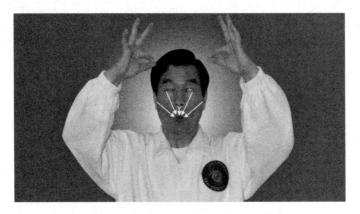

Draw all your energy into your mouth.

8. Exhale, lower your heels to the ground, and relax. Move your tongue around 6–9 times and mix all the energies of the universe with your saliva, but do not swallow it.

9. Repeat steps 2–8 two more times, until you have a mouth full of energized saliva.

10. When you are ready, press all of your fingers around the pinkies, inhale, pull up the middle part of the anus, and press your tongue to the roof of your mouth. On the next inhalation, pull the left and right sides of the anus up toward the left and right kidneys, feeling the kidneys pushing up the tongue.

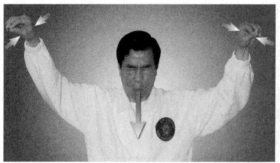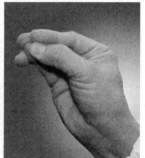

Squeeze the pinkies and swallow.

11. Lock your neck, press your tongue hard against your palate, and squeeze your fingers against your pinkies. Squeeze all the muscles of your body, then swallow all the saliva in one firm gulp, delivering the elixir straight to your stomach. Smile to your organs and feel the chi/saliva/elixir spreading to them.

12. Rest and cover your navel, feeling it grow warm. Guide the chi down the front of your legs to the toes and soles as you sink your body down. Scoop up the Earth Chi with your arms, and then pour it into your crown.

13. Collect energy at your navel.

⟳ Looking Back at the Moon

(Pages 78–80)

1. Stand with your feet together and hands loosely curled. Place the back of your right hand in front of your forehead and the left hand at waist level, palm toward your body.

2. Rotate your spine leftward, looking back over your shoulder toward your right heel. Let your hands move leftward.

3. Gather energy through your armpit hair, then contract your anus, perineum, and genitals. Press your tongue to your palate and hold your breath for 10 seconds. Feel the energy collecting in your hair.

4. Exhale and use your tongue to beat the saliva in your mouth without swallowing it. Repeat steps 1–4 two more times.

5. Squeeze your fists tightly and swallow the elixir firmly down into the navel. Swallow hard 3 times.

6. Repeat the whole exercise with hands reversed, this time turning to the right.

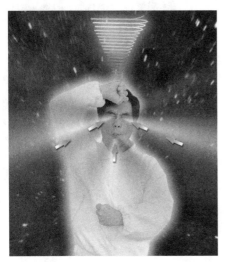

Place right fist at forehead facing out and the left fist at waist level facing in.

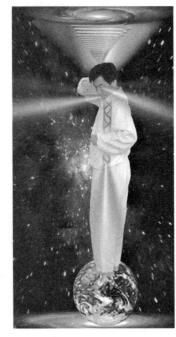

Rotate to the left and look over your shoulder to your right heel.

Looking Back at the Moon

⟳ Wai T'o Offering the Rod

(Pages 81–84)

1. Stand with your feet shoulder-width apart and arms extended out to the sides, palms down. Press your wrists down. Feel your body press down into the earth.
2. Inhale and stretch your fingers toward the sky, stretching the tendons in your hands and forearms.
3. Feel your hair like antennae extended into space. Gather energy

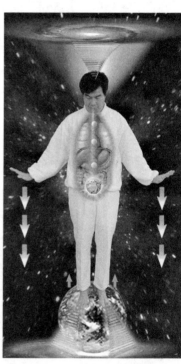

Press the arms down when you swallow.

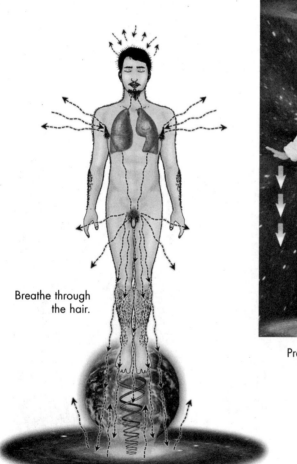

Breathe through the hair.

Wai T'o Offering the Rod

through your head hair and armpit hair while maintaining awareness of your heart and tongue. Then gather energy through the hairs on your arms.

4. Draw energy from your armpits into your mouth: suck on your tongue, draw in your cheeks, and pull your eyes in.

5. Inhale a reverse breath, pulling in the lower abdomen. Feel surplus sexual energy flowing from your pubic hair into your groin. Exhale, feeling the energy exit through your pubic hair.

6. Feel the connection between the pubic hair, lungs, and nose. Breathe through your pubic hair for at least a minute, drawing energy in from the universe. (You may notice some arousal doing this.) Feel the energy from your head hair, armpit hair, arm hair, and pubic hair mixing into your saliva.

7. Draw the energy up toward your mouth: stand on your toes, suck on your tongue, draw in your cheeks, and pull your eyes in. Stretch your palms and fingers upward and draw in more energy.

8. Lower your heels down and feel all the energy from your hair mixing with your saliva. Hold your breath, then exhale and relax your hands.

9. Repeat steps 1–8 three times, then, with arms outstretched, inhale and rise up onto your toes. Pull up your anus and press your tongue to your palate. Press your shoulders, arms, and hands firmly downward and swallow your saliva directly into your navel. Feel the hot saliva and energy press down into your navel.

Giant Raises the Tower
(Pages 84–89)

1. Stand with your feet shoulder-width apart and knees slightly bent. Feel your weight sinking. Curl both hands in loose fists at your waist, palms up.

2. Slowly raise your left palm up past your head, fingers together, then gather the energy of the universe through your armpit hair, feeling the connection to your spleen and mouth.

3. Inhale a reverse breath and feel the energy gathering in your facial

hair. Exhale and feel the energy leaving through your facial hair. Continue breathing through your facial hair for 1 minute.

4. Next, inhale through your facial hair and keep the energy in your mouth when you exhale. Draw in your tongue and cheeks for 30 seconds.

5. Fill your mouth with saliva by swirling your tongue between your front teeth and the backs of your lips—9 times in each direction. Then swirl your tongue behind your front teeth, also 9 times in each direction.

6. Feel the energy from your scalp hair, arm and armpit hair, pubic hair, and facial hair mixing into your saliva. Move your lower jaw as if you were "chewing" the saliva.

7. Breathe through all of your body hair follicles, drawing in universal energy from the six directions around you. Feel the connection between your lungs and nose.

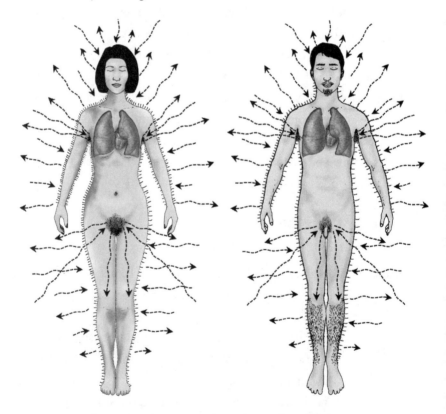

Breathe universal energy in through your hair follicles.

8. Inhale, rise onto your toes, and pull up the middle part of your anus toward your head. Draw in the hair energy by sucking in your cheeks and tongue, pulling your ears toward the ear canals and your eyes toward their sockets. Hold your breath and pull in more tightly, using suction to draw all the energy into your mouth.

9. Exhale and lower your feet to the ground. Inhale Universal Chi, and mix it with the hair energy in your saliva. Repeat steps 1–9 three times, gathering more and more energy into your saliva.

10. Inhale and pull up your anus and tongue. Turn your left upraised hand palm downward to face your body.

11. Swallow hard down into the abdomen as you thrust your left hand down toward the earth. Feel the saliva turn into chi in your navel.

12. Repeat steps 1–11 with hands reversed, then repeat steps 1–11 again with both hands raised.

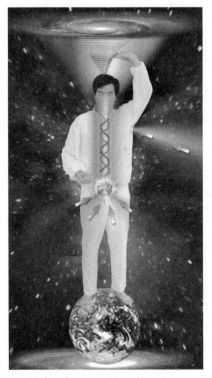 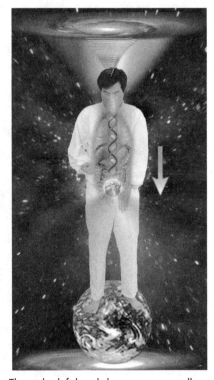

Left palm up, raising the tower   Thrust the left hand down as you swallow.

Giant Raises the Tower

Iron Bridge Swallow

(Pages 90–92)

1. Stand with your feet shoulder-width apart and your ankles locked. Rub your palms together then place them behind your kidneys with the thumbs and index fingers forming a circle on each hand. (Keep the other fingers straight.)
2. Tuck your chin in and bend backward from your lower vertebrae. Do not tip your head backward.

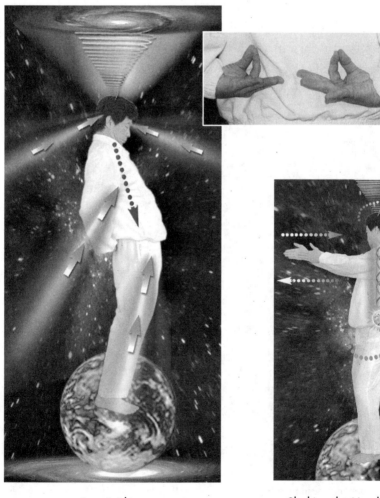

Iron Bridge
Swallow

Shaking the Head and
Wagging the Tail

3. Gather energy from all of your body's hair and senses; draw it into your mouth and saliva as in the previous exercises. Draw in your sense organs, contract your perineum and genitals, and feel the energy collecting in your hair.

4. Inhale and beat the saliva with your tongue. Exhale and relax your face, but do not swallow the saliva. Repeat steps 1–4 two more times.

5. Lightly straighten your neck and press all of your fingers into the pinkies as you swallow hard. Then rest and gently brush the energy down your chest.

🌀 Shaking the Head and Wagging the Tail
(Pages 93–95)

1. Stand with your feet shoulder-width apart and your arms extended forward.

2. All at the same time, do the following: Rub your palms briskly together, waggle your head and your "tail" (sacrum and pelvis) in opposite directions, draw the sense organs into your head, and beat the saliva in your mouth. Continue these movements for 2 minutes.

3. Cover your temples with your warm palms, then cover and massage your face.

4. Cover your upper chest. As you swallow hard, drawing the saliva to your lower tan tien through the chest, heart, belly, and navel, brush your hands downward toward your pelvis. This will rub away the heart's worries.

🌀 Pull the Silk and Swing the Leg
(Pages 95–97)

1. Begin with your right foot one step behind your left and your arms "hugging" the front of your body: place your right hand in front of your left shoulder and your left hand above your right hip.

2. Swing your right leg out in front of you, shifting your weight forward onto your left leg. At the same time, arch your back by pressing your waist and T11 forward, and fling your arms open, straightening your elbows and expanding your chest. Your left palm should be open

toward the sky, your right palm facing the earth. Swing your head to the right, eyes following the downturned palm.

3. Re-cross your arms in front of your body, this time placing your left hand in front of the right shoulder and the right hand above the left hip. Tuck your chin in.

4. Swing your left leg forward, repeating all the motions in step 2 on the opposite side.

5. Repeat each side 50 times.

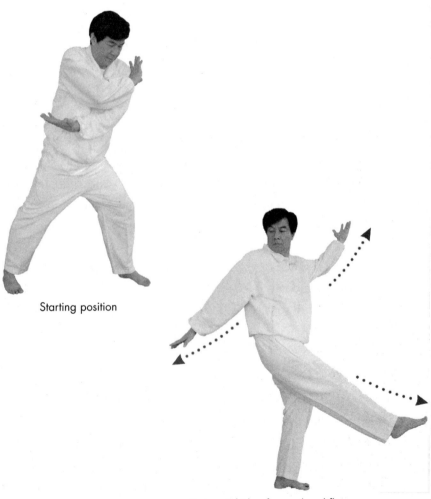

Starting position

Swing right leg forward and fling arms open.

Pull the Silk and Swing the Leg

⟳ Gathering the Golden Earth Pill
(Pages 98–103)

1. On a piece of 8½ × 11-inch paper, draw two 6-inch circles intersecting each other. Draw a dot in the center of the intersecting region.
2. Stand with your feet shoulder-width apart, and place the drawing between your feet. Squat down, letting your buttocks almost touch the ground.
3. Place your hands on your hips and practice rotating your left leg back and forth from the hip—left to right and right to left. Do the same with your right leg, then with both legs together.

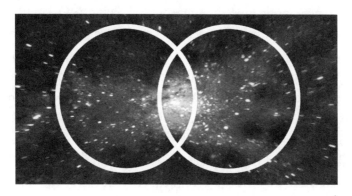

Draw two intersecting circles.

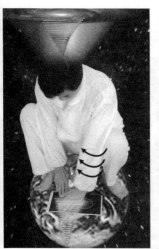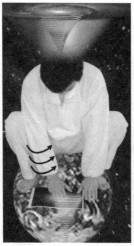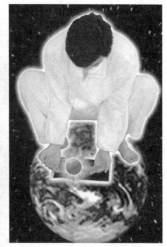

Rotate each hip, pushing the arms to trace two circles.   Scoop up the earth pill.

4. Draw a dot in the center of each palm, then drop your hands down in front of you, locking your elbows and resting them against the insides of your knees.

5. Move your right hip so that your leg pushes your arm: your arm will swing and your palm will trace the right-hand circle in a counterclockwise motion. Do not use the muscles of your hand or arm to trace the circle; just let the hip push your arm around.

6. Do the same with your left hip, pushing your left arm to trace the left-hand circle. Focus your eyes on the dot in the center of the intersecting circles.

7. Now move both hips simultaneously, keeping your circling palms about 1 inch from the paper. At the overlapping point where the hands cross, a pearl of energy is created—this is the "earth pill."

8. Use your mind, eyes, and palms to gather the earth force 3 times. Notice the earth pill forming. At the same time, gather the energy of the senses and organs into your head and saliva.

9. Scoop the earth pill up in your hands as you stand up. Inhale, then suck the earth pill from your hands deep into your mouth. Pull up you anus and mix the earth pill with your saliva.

10. Press your tongue against your palate and beat the saliva, then swallow it down, bringing your cupped palms to face your chest. Feel the saliva and the earth pill rush down to your stomach and lower tan tien as you sweep your hands down your chest.

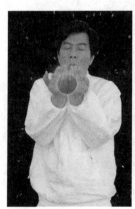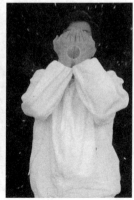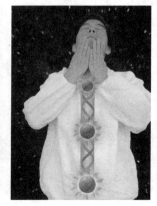

Mix the earth pill with your saliva and swallow.

🌀 Tiger Out of the Cage

(Pages 103–7)

1. Stand with your feet about 3 feet apart and your hands in fists at your waist, facing upward.
2. Punch straight ahead with your right fist, rotating the wrist so the fingers point downward as you punch. At the same time, lower your right knee and shift your weight to the right leg.
3. As a variation, twist your punching arm clockwise as far as you can.
4. At the end of the punch, form a fierce claw with your right hand, spreading and tensing the fingers. Pretend to claw at the eyes of an imaginary assailant, then grasp and twist his nose and mouth clockwise. Grab the beard or chin of your imaginary opponent and pull him toward you to upset his balance. At the same time, shift most of your weight back onto your left leg.
5. Rotate your wrist so the claw is facing upward, then retract it, closing your hand back into a fist and bringing it back to your waist.

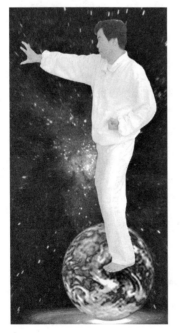

Starting position

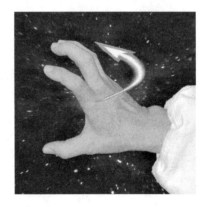

Tiger Out of the Cage

6. Repeat steps 2–5 on the left side, twisting your left arm counterclockwise as you punch.

7. Practice 108 times on each side.

⚙ Iron Buffalo Plows the Land

(Pages 107–9)

1. Stand with your feet 6 inches apart and "walk" your hands forward on the floor. Form a triangle by keeping your knees and elbows straight and your hips high. Begin by supporting your weight on your hands; with practice you will be able to support your weight with your fingertips.

2. Gather energy in your mouth and mix it with your saliva. As you prepare to swallow, bend your arms and scoop your nose forward, about an inch off the ground.

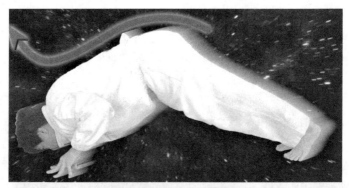

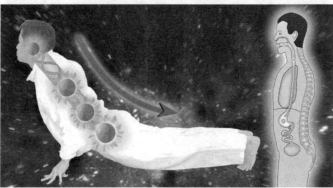

Raise the head like a cobra as you swallow.

Iron Buffalo Plows the Land

3. As you swallow, swing your hips forward and arch your back. As your head rises up, swallow the saliva down.

4. Repeat this exercise 3 times the first month, 6 times the second month, 9 times the third month, and 12 times the fourth month.

⟳ Fair Lady Jumps
(Pages 110–14)

1. Stand upright with your knees straight and feet close together.

2. Swing your arms at your sides and smile to your heart, feeling happy and light throughout your body.

3. When you feel light enough to fly, sink your power into your lower tan tien and toes. Bending your knees and hips only slightly, jump straight upward, thrusting your arms straight up at the same time.

4. Brush congested chi down your chest with your hands. Repeat the jump 9–18 times, then walk around for a few minutes. Never eat, drink, or sit down immediately after jumping.

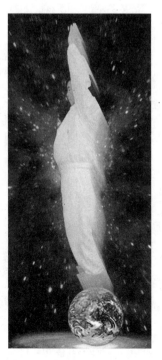

Fair Lady Jumps

🌀 Ending Exercise

Whether you have practiced one or more of the Elixir Chi Kung practices, always complete your session with this exercise.

1. Stand with your feet close together and raise your palms to the heavens. Feel chi from the universe flowing into your hollow bones and compressing there.

2. With very big and long hands, scoop up chi from the universe and pour it over your crown. Feel electricity run into your skull and bones. Brush the energy down your body, then feel your legs sink deep into the center of the earth.

3. Now scoop the Earth Chi from the earth below you. Guide it up the bones of your body.

4. Scoop chi down from the crown again, moving it into your lower tan tien. Cover your navel with your hands and collect the energy there.

5. Rest by brushing your hands down your chest and walking around.

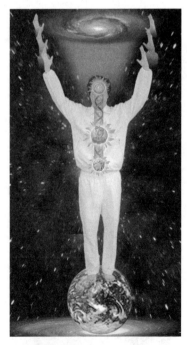

Ending exercise: gathering
and scooping the chi

TAI CHI FA JIN

Opening Movements

(Pages 114–20)

1. Stand facing north with your feet together and your head suspended from a string connected to the heavenly force. Sink down, then smile from the eyes down to the navel. Inhale while rounding the scapulae, sinking the chest, and opening the armpits. Then exhale while sinking down.

2. Shift your tailbone to the right heel and lift the left heel up. Inhale while picking up your left foot, then exhale as you set the left foot down a shoulder-width apart, at a 30-degree angle. Maintain basic Iron Shirt posture with the left foot open.

3. Shift your tailbone over the left heel. Draw your right hip forward, then step with the right foot and reach with the right hand facing north.

4. Draw your right hip and arm back while simultaneously moving the left hip and hand forward. Shift your tailbone to left heel and sink back.

5. Turn left, and torque your left hip while bringing your left forearm up to protect your head. Let the movement of your hips turn your right foot 90 degrees, then shift tailbone to left heel.

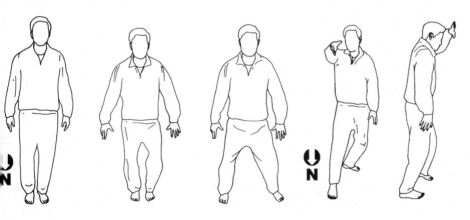

Left-Hand Form: opening the form

⟳ First Corner, South (Left-Hand Form)
(Pages 120–27)

1. Turn hips to left, then shift tailbone to right heel. Step wide on left toes, facing south. Raise your right hand from the right hip, circling with the left hand twice, then forming a chi ball.

2. Ward Off Strike: Sink back–kick left foot back–discharge forward wide–drag stiff right leg (anchor leg)–right foot straight–no upper movement–sink back.

3. Rollback: Turn hips to right, facing west–drop right hand to left elbow–eyes focus on left palm.

4. Press Strike: Outer right wrist connects to inner left wrist–kick left foot back–discharge forward wide–drag right foot straight (anchor leg)–no upper movement.

5. Push Strike: Sink back–separate wrists–open palms–kick left foot back–discharge forward wide–drag stiff right foot straight (anchor leg)–no upper movement.

6. Single Whip: Sink back–turn hips to right facing west–form right hand beak over left palm–weight on right.

7. Prepare Lady Shuttle: Sink back–step left heel to south–turn left foot 90 degrees west while dropping left hand to protect left knee. Shift

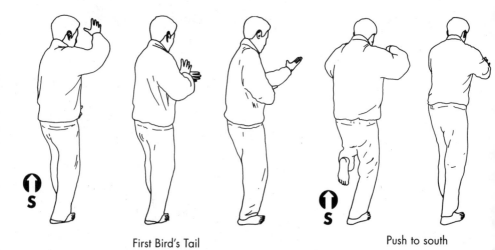

First Bird's Tail

Push to south

Left-Hand Form: first corner to the south

tailbone to left heel–right foot step wide to right facing north–circle right hand with left hand twice to right forming chi ball–weight on left foot.

8. Lady Shuttle Strike: Sink back–strike–push left hand forward with hip–roll right hand up to protect head–facing north.

9. Change directions: Step back with left foot pointing west–open hip to west–draw right hand down (crossing left wrist) protecting right knee. Left hand protects head–shift tailbone to left heel–left hand down to left knee and right hand up to protect head. Shift tailbone to right heel–circle hands twice forming chi ball facing west.

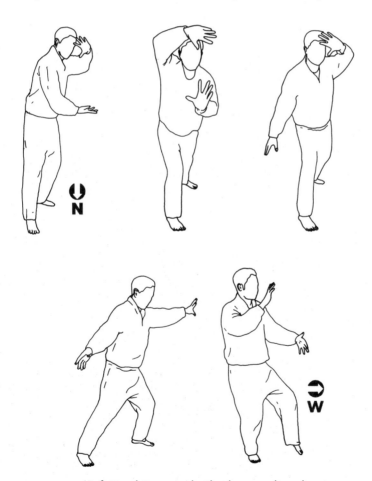

Left-Hand Form: Lady Shuttle to north and
transition to second corner (west)

✪ Second Corner (West), Left-Hand Form
(Pages 125–27)

1. Form chi ball.
2. Ward Off: Sink back–kick left foot back–discharge to west, forward and wide–drag stiff right leg (anchor leg)–right foot straight–no upper movement–sink back.
3. Rollback.
4. Press: Same footwork as Ward Off–strike with connecting wrists.
5. Push: Sink back–separate wrists–open palms–kick left foot back–discharge forward (west) wide–drag stiff right foot straight–no upper movement.
6. Single Whip: Sink back–turn hips to right facing north–form right hand beak over left palm–weight on right leg.
7. Lady Shuttle to the east: Step left heel to west–turn left foot 90 degrees north while dropping left hand to protect left knee–shift tailbone to left heel–right foot step wide to right (facing east)–circle right hand with left hand twice to right–form chi ball.
8. Sink back–strike–push left hand forward with hip–roll right hand up protecting head.
9. Change directions: Step back with left foot pointing north–open hip to north while drawing right hand down (crossing left wrist) to protect right knee–left hand protecting head–shift tailbone to left heel–left hand down to left knee and right hand up protecting head.

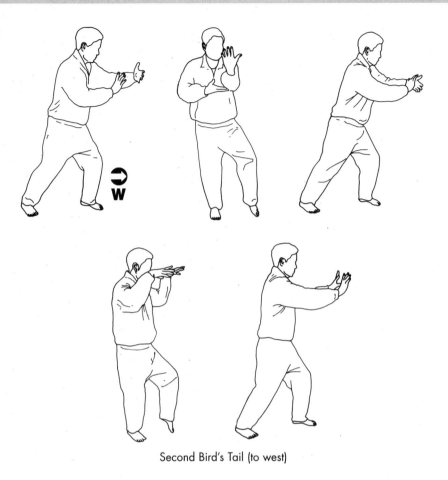

Second Bird's Tail (to west)

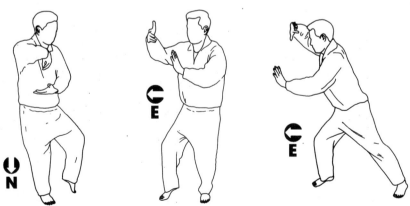

Single Whip, then Lady Shuttle to the east

Left-Hand Form: second corner to the west

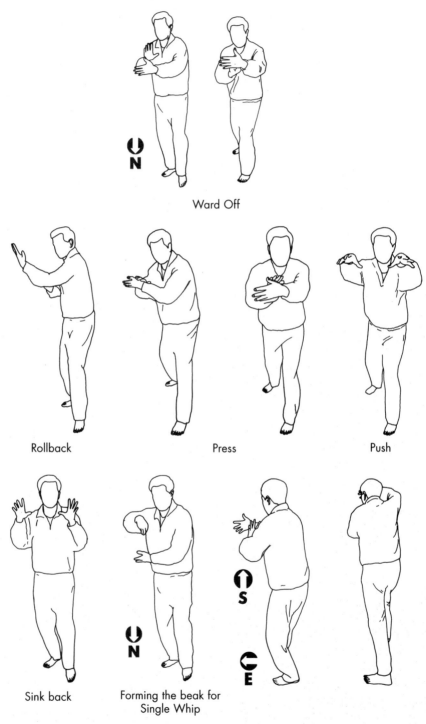

Ward Off

Rollback   Press   Push

Sink back   Forming the beak for
Single Whip

Left-Hand Form: third corner to the north

⚙ North, East, and South Corners (Left-Hand Form)

(Pages 128–34)

1. Shift tailbone to right heel–circle hands twice–form chi ball facing north.
2. Ward Off–Rollback–Press–Push–Single Whip–Lady Shuttle–Changing Directions.
3. Repeat steps 1 and 2 to the east corner, then repeat them again to the south corner.

⚙ Transition to Right-Hand Form

(Pages 133–41)

After the transition to the right-hand form in step 1 below, the movements progress in a counterclockwise direction and strikes are performed with the right hand.

1. Step left foot forward–shift tailbone to left heel–draw left hand forward and right hand back–shift tailbone to right heel–left hand to left hip and right hand forward–turn hips 90 degrees to right (face south)–right foot pointing east–right arm protects head–shift tailbone to left heel–weight on left foot.

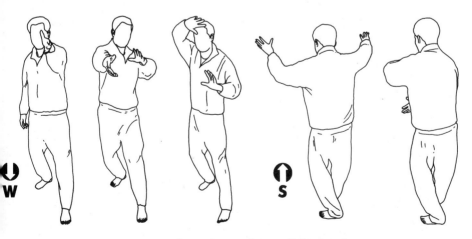

Transition to the Right-Hand Form (following the fifth corner of the Left-Hand Form)

2. Right foot steps wide to right (facing south)–circle right hand around left hand twice to right–form chi ball.

3. Ward Off Strike: Sink back–kick right foot back–discharge forward wide–drag stiff left leg (anchor leg) left foot straight–no upper movement.

4. Rollback–Press–Push–Single Whip–Lady Shuttle–Changing Directions.

5. Repeat steps 2–4 for the east corner, the north corner, the west corner, then the south corner again.

Completion

(Page 142)

1. After releasing Lady Shuttle, open both hands. Move them up and outward then downward, drawing the left foot straight back setting it down parallel to the right foot. Shift tailbone to left heel–lift up right leg placing it parallel with left–draw feet together with toes even.

2. Raise hands 12 inches in front of body, then cross right wrist over left wrist and place them on your chest to form an X below the shoulders.

3. Distribute weight evenly between both feet. Simultaneously straighten body and lower hands to sides, with palms facing back. All movement ends at same time. Relax and center yourself, and feel the chi expand in your body.

4. Smile down, and collect energy at your navel.

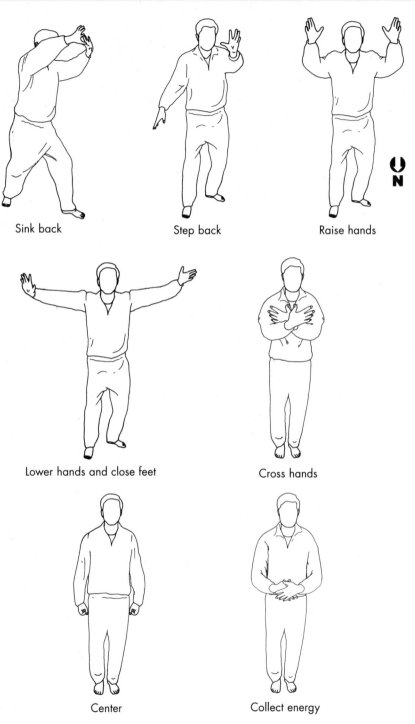

Sink back

Step back

Raise hands

Lower hands and close feet

Cross hands

Center

Collect energy

Closing the form

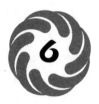

Level Six

The sixth level of the Universal Healing Tao system consists of over forty formulas that can be found in the Destiny Books editions of these Universal Healing Tao books: *The Taoist Soul Body, Karsai Nei Tsang,* and *Tai Chi Wu Style.*

At this level we begin to give birth: first to the soul and then to the spirit in the body. The body has been developed to become a fit dwelling place for the soul and spirit, and it must also provide nourishment through the energies accumulated through the beginning practices. Giving birth to the soul is awakening that part of ourselves that perceives and acts free from environmental, educational, and karmic conditioning. Gaining awareness through the awakened soul to be creatively active in the world, we learn to not merely react to circumstances. This level of meditation has many physiological effects as well, further preparing the body to accommodate the greater amounts of energy necessary for the birth and nourishment of soul and spirit.

THE TAOIST SOUL BODY: HARNESSING THE POWER OF KAN AND LI

Theory: The meditations of the Lesser, Greater, and Greatest Enlightenment of Kan and Li lead to the birth of the soul and the spirit in the body, as well as to the formation of the immortal spirit body. At this stage of practice, the energies of nature (the sun, the moon, the trees, etc.) and practically all sensory experiences of a positive nature become palatable nourishment for the growth and maturing of the spirit in the body. The formulas of Lesser Kan and Li use darkness technology to literally steam the sexual energy (ching) into life-force energy (chi) by reversing the location of yin and yang power. This creates an internal energetic streaming machine, which is required for the final transformation of the Inner Alchemy practices.

Concept: This inversion places the heat of the fire from the heart center beneath the coolness of the water generated by the sexual energy of the perineum, thereby activating the liberation of transformed sexual energy. Darkness technology has been a key element of this practice and of all Inner Alchemy traditions throughout the ages. The darkness actualizes successively higher states of consciousness, correlating with the accumulation of psychedelic chemicals in the brain. In the darkness, mind and soul begin to wander freely in the vast realms of psychic and spiritual experience.

Through these practices, we awaken to that which is eternal and enduring behind the appearances of sensory information. Aware of our true nature as spirit, we experience a self beyond the cycle of life and death.

Purpose: The birth of the soul is not a metaphor. It is an actual process of converting energy into a subtle body (spaceship) to travel beyond time and space. Developing the soul body is the preparation for the growth of the immortal spirit body in the practice of the Greater Enlightenment of Kan and Li. In the final stage of this practice, the adept unites spirit, soul, and body, or separates them at will. The human being then knows full and complete freedom.

KARSAI NEI TSANG

Theory: Karsai Nei Tsang is the third level of the Chi Nei Tsang practices of the Universal Healing Tao. It focuses on the blockages in the genital area, especially those that take the form of sedimentation in the blood vessels. When the genitals suffer from blockages, the Ching Chi (sexual chi) is not free to circulate through the body, which is then deprived of this powerful healing energy.

Concept: Our sexual organs play a major role in our physical and emotional health. Many emotional traumas and stresses are stored in the pelvic region in the form of tension—in the muscles, ligaments, and tendons—and imbalances in the meridians and organs, resulting in an accumulation of toxins and energetic knots and tangles. By freeing the Ching Chi of the sexual organs through massage, meridian clearing, and detoxification, Karsai Nei Tsang helps to resolve physical and emotional blockages in the pelvic area.

Purpose: Because blockages and sedimentations tend to manifest around age forty, Karsai Nei Tsang is especially important for men and women over the age of forty, as well as and for anyone who feels blocked sexually. Karsai Nei Tsang addresses common problems associated with our sexual organs, such as impotence, frequent and difficult urination, painful menstruation, painful intercourse, and low sexual libido. It is also quite effective in alleviating lower back pain, improving the body's alignment, strengthening the pelvic floor muscles, and increasing general vitality.

TAI CHI WU STYLE

Theory: This practice is the Tai Chi Chi Kung Wu Style Form of the Universal Healing Tao. It begins in the north, moves counterclockwise 360 degrees, and then returns clockwise 360 degrees. This Short Wu Style Form highlights some of the essential movements taken from the Long Wu form. Practitioners may perform the Tai Chi Chi Kung Wu Style form in an abbreviated version to three directions or in an expanded version to eight directions.

Concept: The beginner learns the sequence initially with the intellectual mind and gradually comes to embody the underlying principles. Over time, the student learns to integrate the form with the principles of Tan Tien Chi Kung and Iron Shirt practice, as well as with the breath, martial applications, and spirit. Once you learn the form, you will know it completely, activating your molecular memory.

Purpose: By practicing the Tai Chi forms daily, you enforce the movements in your energy body, which is what you will take with you to the next realm: its postures and strikes will be part of your dense spaceship energetic yang body. In this form, you will learn anatomical and geographical placement of your body, as well as movements for opening up your tendons and expanding your body strength with the spirit aspects of the form.

THE TAOIST SOUL BODY
Defining Kan and Li

Kan: Life Essence, Orgasmic Energy
(Pages 8–17)

- Lead: dense and heavy. The white tiger's energy relates to metal and the lungs.
- True sense/True Lead = real knowledge; when sexual energy cannot be moved the senses will be restored.
- True sense is outwardly dark but inwardly bright: strong and unbending, yang within yin, able to ward off external afflictions. The black tiger's strength and vigor are within.
- The North Star conceals brightness within darkness and metal within water.

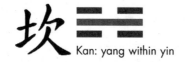
Kan: yang within yin

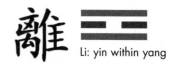
Li: yin within yang

THE CHARACTERISTICS OF KAN AND LI

Kan	Li
Water	Fire
Lead, true sense, endurance, stamina	Mercury, spiritual essence, virtue
Sexual energy	Compassionate energy
Yang within yin	Yin within yang
Lady of the Kan in the Moon	Maiden of the Li in the Sun
North, Moon	South, Sun
White tiger	Green dragon
Female	Male
Kidney	Heart
Saliva	Chi
Semen, sperm	Blood, menstruation
Black	Red
Self	Other
True sense mixed with arbitrary feeling	Spiritual essences are adulterated with temper

- Rabbit in the Moon—masculinity within femininity.
- When sexual energy rises (does not leak out) it transforms into bliss.
- Total body multi-orgasm: first brain, then senses, then kidneys, then liver, then spleen, then lungs, then heart, then soul, then spirit.
- The orgasm comes from the material substances: the sexual organs, the senses, the glands, the organs.
- Aroused sexual energy can be transformed into the immaterial—the Ching Chi.
- When aroused to a higher level, the multi-orgasm has the power to connect with universal force (God) and bring earth energy up to the human body.

Li: Spiritual Essence, Heart Compassion Fire

- Mercury: lively and active, bright and buoyant. It flows easily in the human body. The green dragon's energy is related to wood.
- Spiritual essence/True Mercury is outwardly firm yet inwardly flexible. Call and it responds; touch and it moves. True Mercury goes in and out unpredictably.
- When it is passing through or being tempered by fire, the green dragon changes to the black tiger (True Lead).
- Women are yin on the outside and yang on the inside; men are yang on the outside and yin on the inside.
- Raven in the Sun—femininity within masculinity.
- Mercury within cinnabar—its reality is hidden within fire.
- Flowing pearl—its light is penetrating.
- The fire of the heart's compassion transforms the material into the immaterial.
- The material—the organs of the heart, kidneys, liver, spleen, lungs—is transformed into the immaterial—the virtues of love, joy, happiness, gentleness, kindness, fairness, and courage. We cannot see or touch these immaterial virtues, but we can feel them.
- When all of these virtues combine at the heart, they become the heart of compassion fire; when they rise up to the mid-eyebrow, they become the spiritual essence.

THE TAOIST SOUL BODY
Lesser Kan and Li Formulas

⚙ Coupling: Reversal of the Hot and Cold Energies
(Pages 91–95)

1. Smile down to the organs. Listen to the kidneys; feel their gentleness and coolness. Distinguish the kidneys' cool energy from the hot energy of the adrenal glands.

2. Become aware of your perineum and sexual energy. Form a spherical collection point at the perineum and begin to collect the cold kidney energy there. Melt the glacier in the perineum into water.

3. Imagine yourself as a god or goddess making love, and collect multiorgasmic energy.

4. Become aware of your heart; spiral chi within it. Feel the radiance of appreciation and the combination of ultraviolet light, infrared light, and good virtue energy blending together into a compassion fire.

5. Become of aware of the powerful adrenal glands storing ultraviolet light like a volcanic fire under the sea. Collect the hot energy of the adrenals at T11, then send it up the spinal cord to the crown. Next, bring it down the Middle Thrusting Channel to the heart center, and combine it with the compassion energies of the heart and thymus.

6. Slowly draw the hot energies from the adrenals, heart, and thymus into the heart's collection point and establish a pulse there.

7. Divide your attention between the hot and cold energies at the two collection points. Without spilling, bring the hot energy down the Left Thrusting Channel to the lower abdomen and the cold energy through the Right Thrusting Channel up the back to the solar plexus.

8. Move the hot and cold energies into the Middle Thrusting Channel and carefully couple them at the navel. The hot energy/fire is the stove, and the cold energy/water is the cauldron.

9. Establish a heartbeat in the cauldron and allow the kidneys to pulse along with it as you pull up sexual energy. Feel the Earth pulsing in synchrony. Seal your senses into the cauldron to maintain the automatic pulse there.

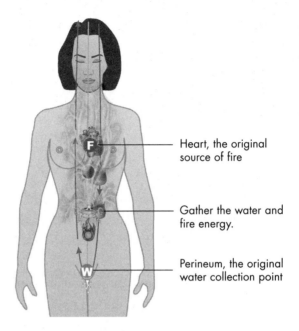

Heart, the original source of fire

Gather the water and fire energy.

Perineum, the original water collection point

Gathering the water and fire energies

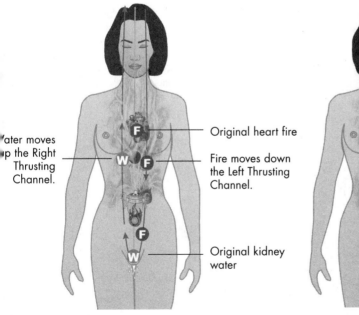

Water moves up the Right Thrusting Channel.

Original heart fire

Fire moves down the Left Thrusting Channel.

Original kidney water

Move fire to the center of the lower abdomen. Move water to the solar plexus.

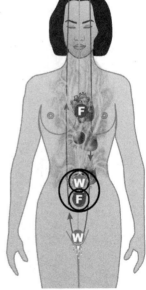

Couple water and fire at the navel.

10. Breathe gently into the cauldron, feeling the ultraviolet light cooking all the atoms together. Stir the cauldron with your inner eye and feel the steam rise.

11. Feel the sacred water and orgasm energy rise from the coccyx to the sacrum and then to T11; pour it into the cauldron.

❷ Steaming the Five Vital Organs
(Pages 96–98)

1. Become aware of the steaming cauldron. Smile into your kidneys and direct the steam into them. Steam and gently cook the kidneys, feeling a blue fragrance blow out of them, removing toxins, bad genes, and sick energy.

2. Smile to the liver and gallbladder and direct the steam into them until they are rid of toxins, bad genes, and sick energy.

3. Repeat for the spleen, pancreas, and stomach, the heart and small intestine, and the lungs and large intestine.

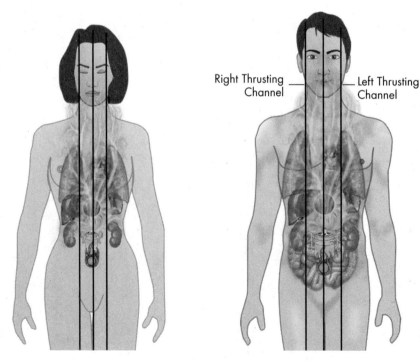

Right Thrusting Channel   Left Thrusting Channel

Steaming the five vital organs

⚙ Steaming the Endocrine Glands
(Pages 98–100)

1. Smile down to your thymus gland (the "virtue gland") and direct steam into it, allowing it to regenerate. Send two-thirds of the available steam into your thymus, and divide the remaining one-third among the other glands.
2. Steam the thyroid, parathyroid, and salivary glands inside the throat.
3. Turn your eyes to the mid-eyebrow point and direct steam into your pituitary gland.
4. Turn your eyes up to the top of your head and steam your pineal gland.
5. Focus on the center of your brain and steam your hypothalamus.
6. Steam your adrenal glands and sexual organs.

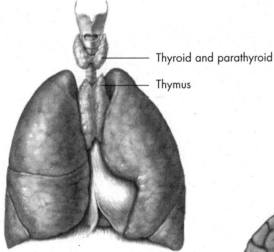

Thyroid and parathyroid

Thymus

Steaming the thyroid,
parathyroid, and thymus gland

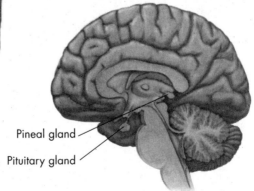

Pineal gland

Pituitary gland

Steaming the endocrine glands

⟳ Steaming the Spine, Lymphatic System, and Nerves

(Pages 100, 102, 120)

1. Stir the cauldron and pull up your sexual organs with your eyes. Feel the energy pushing the cauldron and stove back toward your spine.
2. Direct the steam into your spine. Breathe the energy up and down

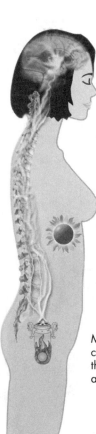

Move the cauldron into the lower spinal area.

Steaming the spinal cord

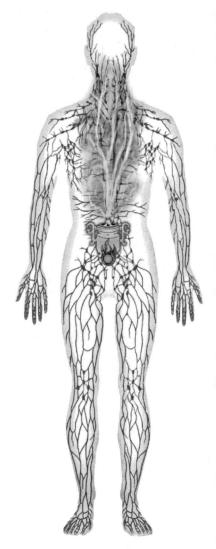

Steaming the lymphatic system

your spine, letting it clean, repair, and regenerate the spinal cord and spinal fluid.

3. Direct the steam into the lymph nodes in the navel area; feel them opening one by one. Then direct the steam to lymph nodes in the chest, neck, armpits, arms, hands, groin, legs, and feet. Let the steam clean, repair, and regenerate the whole lymphatic system.

4. Move the stove and cauldron carefully down to your perineum, then up into the sacrum. From there, steam your spinal cord. Let the steam fill the spinal cord, then flow out of it into the nerves throughout the body. Focus on moistening dry areas and the nerve endings. Feel the steam cleaning, repairing, and regenerating your entire nervous system.

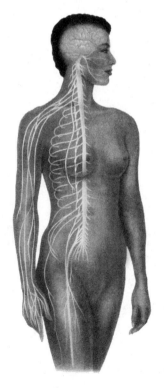

Steaming the nervous system

THE TAOIST SOUL BODY
Opening and Steaming the Twelve Organ Meridians

For the following practices, you will need to locate the ching-well points at the lower corners of the finger- and toenails. With the palms (or soles) down, the *medial* side refers to the side nearest the thumb (or big toe), while the *lateral* side is nearer the pinkie.

As you finish steaming each channel, remember that the next channel begins very nearby. Make a mental connection to the next channel as you shift to its holding point.

Steaming Lung and Large Intestine Channels
(Pages 103–5)

1. Reestablish the pulse at the cauldron and place the tips of your index fingers on the holding points for the lungs: the outer bottom corner

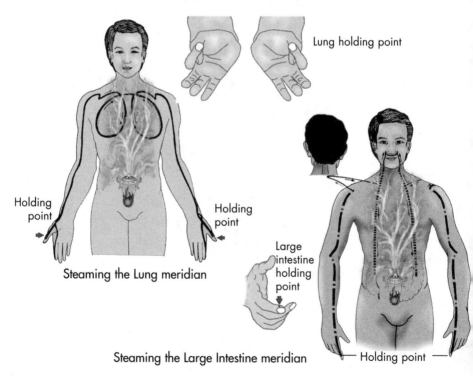

Lung holding point

Holding point

Holding point

Steaming the Lung meridian

Large intestine holding point

Steaming the Large Intestine meridian

Holding point

of your thumbnails. Steam the lungs and the Lung meridians, mentally tracing the channels.

2. Hold the large intestine points by placing the tips of your thumbs on the medial side of the index fingers, at the bottom corner of the nail. Steam the large intestine and the Large Intestine meridian.

Steaming the Stomach and Spleen Channels

(Pages 106–8)

1. Hold the lung points with your fingers as you focus your inner eye on the stomach holding points: the lower lateral corner of the second toenail. Steam the stomach and the Stomach meridians, mentally tracing the channels.

2. Hold the lung points with your fingers as you focus your mental energy on the spleen holding points: the inner edge of the big toe, at the lower corner of the nail. Steam the spleen and the Spleen meridians.

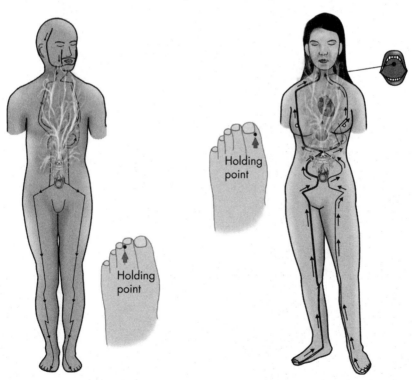

Steaming the Stomach meridian   Steaming the Spleen meridian

✿ Steaming the Heart and Small Intestine Channels

1. Hold the heart points by placing the tips of your thumbs on the medial edge of your pinkie finger, at the lower corner of the nail. Steam the heart and the Heart meridian.
2. Press your thumbs against the lateral edge of the pinkie finger, at the lower corner of the nail. Steam the small intestine and the Small Intestine meridians.

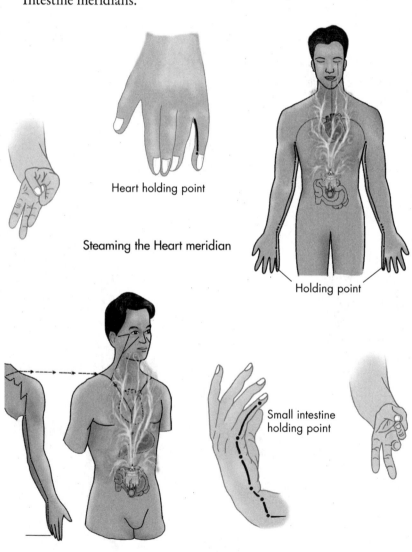

Heart holding point

Steaming the Heart meridian

Holding point

Small intestine holding point

Steaming the Small Intestine meridian

☺ Steaming the Bladder and Kidney Channels

(Pages 110–13)

1. Hold the points at the outer edge of the pinkie toe, at the lower corner of the nail—or focus mentally on these points as you hold the lung points. Gently steam the bladder and the Urinary Bladder meridians, repairing and rejuvenating them.

2. Focus on the holding points for the kidneys—in the center of the soles—as you physically hold the lung points. Steam the kidneys and the Kidney meridians.

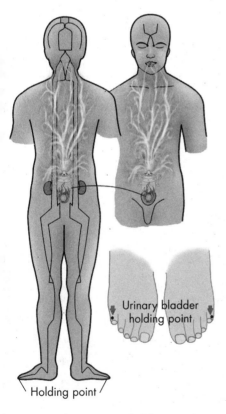

Urinary bladder holding point

Holding point

Steaming the Urinary Bladder meridian

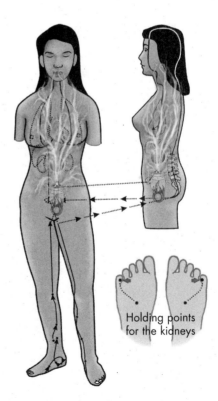

Holding points for the kidneys

Steaming the Kidney meridian

⚙ Steaming the Pericardium and Triple Warmer Channels

(Pages 113–15)

1. Place your thumbs on the tips of your middle fingers and steam the area around the heart. Then steam the Pericardium channels.
2. Place your thumbs on the tips of your ring fingers and steam the upper torso, middle torso, and lower abdomen. Then steam the Triple Warmer meridians.

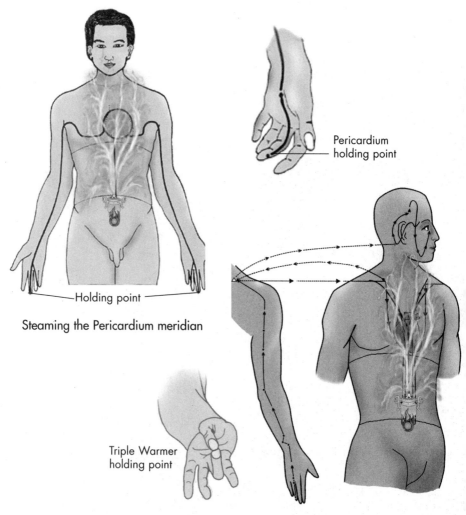

Pericardium holding point

Holding point

Steaming the Pericardium meridian

Triple Warmer holding point

Steaming the Triple Warmer meridian

⟳ Steaming the Gall Bladder and Liver Channels

(Pages 115–17)

1. As you hold the lung points, focus your mind on the gallbladder holding points, located on the lateral edge of the fourth toe, outside the lower corner of the nail. Steam the gallbladder and the Gall Bladder meridians.

2. Hold the lung points and focus your mind on the holding points for the liver, located on the medial edge of the big toes, outside the lower corner of the nail. Steam the liver and the Liver meridians.

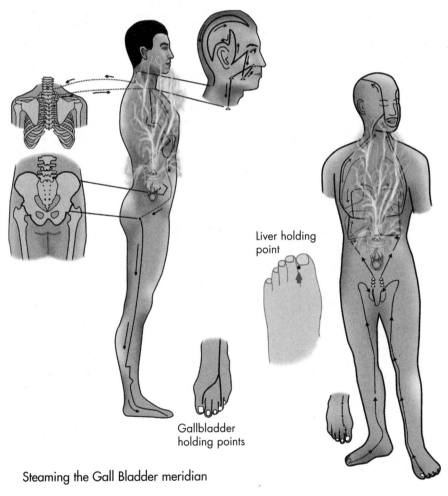

Liver holding point

Gallbladder holding points

Steaming the Gall Bladder meridian

Steaming the Liver meridian

THE TAOIST SOUL BODY
Completing the Lesser Kan and Li Practice

🌀 Increasing the Pulse

(Pages 101–2)

1. Mentally allow the heart rate to decrease.
2. Direct the steam to the aorta and vena cava and feel it pulse there.
3. Move your hand to gently touch the navel and feel the pulse. This will help assist the heart by moving the blood and chi through the groin and inner ankles.
4. Move your hand to very gently touch the neck, temple, back of the skull, armpits, inside elbows, and wrists; amplify the pulse.
5. As you become familiar with this exercise, begin to synchronize all pulses. By recreating the pulse in other areas, you will eventually be able to transfer the heartbeat up to the energy body.

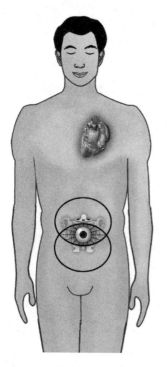

The inner eye

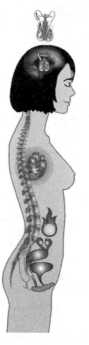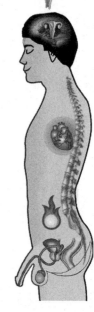

Self-intercourse: the pineal gland is the second sexual organ

☯ The Inner Eye
(Page 121)

1. In the junction point between the stove and cauldron, make the inner eye. You may begin with it as a point of light.
2. Allow the eye to grow and strengthen and begin to move it out of the stove/cauldron.
3. Eventually begin to direct the inner eye on exploratory missions throughout the various routes: the Microcosmic Orbit, Thrusting Channels, etc.

☯ Self-Intercourse
(Pages 122–24)

1. Concentrating on the sexual organs and the pineal gland, practice the Power Lock for several rounds to draw sexual energy up to the pineal gland.*
2. Draw sexual energy into the perineum.
3. Using the Middle Thrusting Channel, feel the connection between the genitals through the perineum and the pineal gland.
4. Draw sexual energy up from the perineum as you bring down energy from the pineal gland, compressing them both into the cauldron at the navel. As you establish their connection at the cauldron, a sexual intensity may occur in the navel area extending out to the organs.
5. When the orgasmic energy reaches what feels to be its peak, seed the cauldron with energy from the liver or the liver collection point. The liver is said to hold the seed of the immortal fetus.

☯ Closing Practice: Turning the Wheel
(Pages 124–25)

Each Kan and Li meditation should be ended with this formula, which is a process of collecting refined energy in the navel cauldron to be used in future meditations, including the higher levels.

---

*For details on the Power Lock, see *Bone Marrow Nei Kung* (Rochester, Vt.: Destiny Books, 2006).

1. Form a pool of sexual energy at the perineum. Looking straight ahead with your eyes closed, form a mental image of a clock with your eyes focused on its center.

2. Look down into the pool (6:00), and draw sexual energy up into the spine. The steam will travel up the spine, drawing sexual energy with it.

3. Look from the perineum up to the right (3:00), drawing the energy up to T11 where it is refined.

4. Look from the right up to the crown (12:00), and draw the energy there to further refine it at the pineal gland.

5. Look from the crown down to the left (9:00), and draw the energy down either through the tongue or the Thrusting Channels into the cauldron at the navel. Store the energy in the cauldron.

6. Repeat steps 2–5 at least 36 times. The rising steam will eventually flow independently of your counting. However, maintain the mental revolutions to be sure it reaches the cauldron.

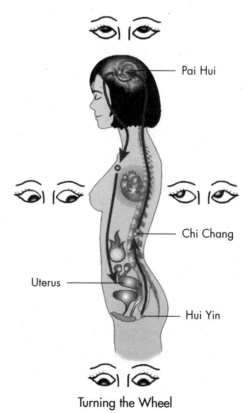

Turning the Wheel

THE TAOIST SOUL BODY
Supplementary Kan and Li Practices

Connecting with the Big Dipper

(Pages 127–31)

According to the Chinese clock, each two hours is one time period, and the stars of the Big Dipper preside over each period (see figures on page 350).

1. **Dubhe—Hungry Wolf/Bright Yang: 11:00 p.m.–1:00 a.m.** Inhale purple light into the cerebellum, then hold your breath and condense the energy. Exhale and observe.

2. **Merak—Huge Gate/Yin Essence: 1:00–3:00 (a.m. and p.m.).** Inhale dark blue light into the memory center. Hold your breath and condense the energy, then exhale.

3. **Phecda—Pure Person/Prosperity Storage: 3:00–5:00 (a.m. and p.m.).** Inhale light blue light into the pineal gland, and condense it there as you hold your breath. Exhale and observe.

4. **Megrez—Intellectual Art/Mystic Subtlety: 5:00–7:00 (a.m. and p.m.).** Inhale green light into the thalamus gland, and condense it there as you hold your breath. Exhale and observe.

5. **Alioth—Honest Chastity/Prime Elixir: 7:00–9:00 (a.m. and p.m.).** Inhale yellow light into the hypothalamus and pituitary gland, and condense the light in these organs as you hold your breath. Exhale and observe.

6. **Mizar—Martial Art/North Pole: 9:00–11:00 (a.m. and p.m.).** Inhale orange light into the olfactory gland, first cranial nerve, and the temples. Condense the light in these areas as you hold your breath, then exhale and observe.

7. **Alcor—Destructive Army/Heavenly Guard: 11:00 a.m.–1:00 p.m.** Inhale red light—the solar fire—into the third eye point, and condense it there as you hold your breath. Exhale and observe.

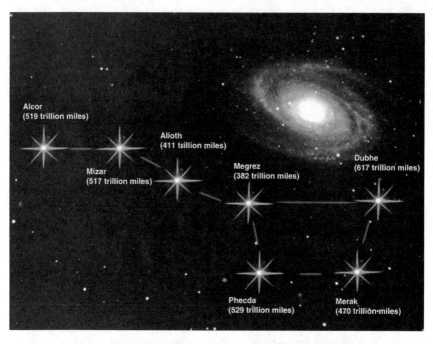

The seven stars of the Big Dipper: Western names and distance from Earth

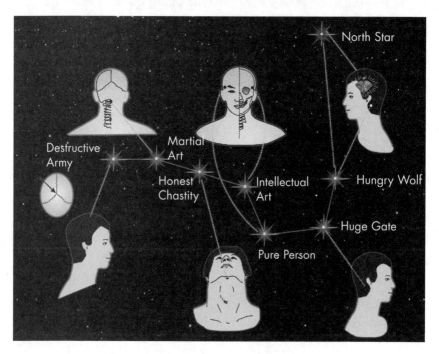

Soul names of the stars in the Big Dipper

☯ Nine Palaces Practice

(Pages 132–44)

1. Let the yin third eye look downward to connect the vocal cords to the thyroid and parathyroid glands; the distance between them is about 7 inches.

2. Inhale and let the true vocal cord generate the green color while the false vocal cord produces the purple color.

3. While sustaining the breath, let your mind gather the condensed vibrations at the corresponding five palaces: the fifth palace connects to the kidneys' sound, the fourth to the liver's sound, the third to the heart's sound, the second to the spleen's sound, and the first to the lungs' sound.

4. Exhale, connecting the sonic vibration from the five organs to the four tones of the four upper palaces; then the tones are allowed to vibrate through the left and right brain. Connecting the left brain to the blue color and the right brain to the purple color connects the power of the moon (left brain) and the sun (right brain).

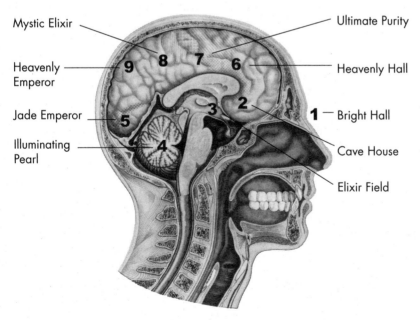

Nine palaces

🌀 Animal Protection Practice (Gathering the Small Pill)
(Pages 144–47)

The Taoist practice involving animal protection consists of calling in the power of each animal to its corresponding organ. There is also a planet acting as a protector of each animal/organ/direction. You can call its power into your chi field by thinking and visualizing, drawing the energy toward you.

1. **Kidneys (black turtle/Mercury):** Place it in the back (north).
2. **Heart (red pheasant/Mars):** Place it in the front (south).
3. **Liver (green dragon/Jupiter):** Place it to the left (east).
4. **Lungs (white tiger/Venus):** Place it on the right (west).
5. **Spleen (yellow phoenix/Saturn):** Place it above your head.
6. When you see a light with your eyes closed, bring it to the cauldron at the navel. Pull up your sexual organs. The light may be dim at first and look like a cloud; it may appear in the middle of the sky or start at the navel and come up to the eyes. You can make it grow brighter. Feel the light inside and outside. Create a pakua in the navel, crown, third eye, or anywhere you wish, even in the palms of the hands or the soles of the feet.
7. Condense the light through the pakua. The bright light will disappear and reappear condensed in the cauldron.
8. Spiral the light in the cauldron and condense it into a pearl. The pearl, the distillation of the external and internal forces, becomes a thick energy ball.
9. Move the pearl down to the perineum and then to the Door of Life (Ming Men) and to the crown. Stop at the crown for about 5 minutes. Then move the pearl down to the solar plexus and into the cauldron at the navel.

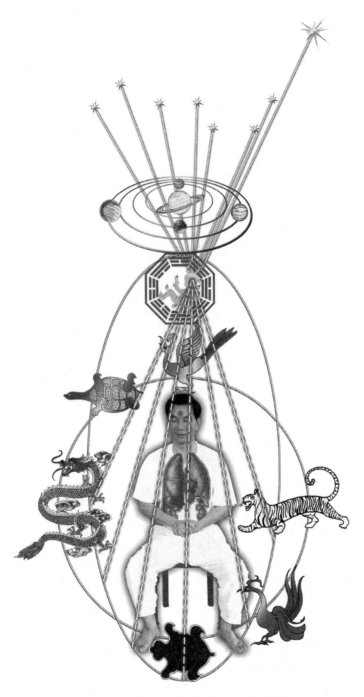

Five sacred animals (Gathering the Pill)

KARSAI NEI TSANG

⟳ Opening the Abdomen

(Pages 36–40)

For the following massages, the student lies in a supine position and the practitioner sits or stands to the side.

1. Scoop with palms around the abdominal perimeter, beginning in the lower right quadrant and moving clockwise. Release any blockages with your Yi–tan tien–universe connection.

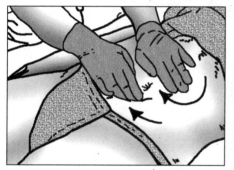 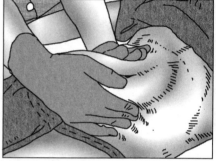

Massaging the abdomen in circles   Kneading the abdomen from side to side

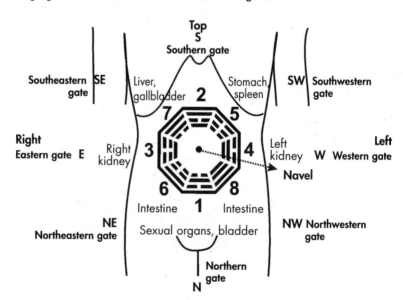

Opening the Wind Gates on the abdominal pakua

2. Knead the abdomen from side to side: Standing on the student's right, use your finger pads to pull up on the descending colon. Use your palms to push the ascending colon in toward the midline. Repeat this rhythmic movement several times.

3. Release specific blockages: Use both thumbs to press in on any areas of sedimentation. Then slowly press both palms into the depth of the restriction until you feel the chi flow returning.

☸ Opening the Wind Gates
(Pages 41–42)

1. Place your right fingers directly below the navel and your left hand over your right.

2. Press in with your finger pads to the level of tension, then pull slightly away from the navel until you feel the tissue softening.

3. Work on the wind gates in order, remembering to pull the tissue outward, away from the navel.

☸ Releasing the Aorta and Inferior Vena Cava
(Pages 42–43)

1. Locate the tan tien point in the depression approximately 1.5 inches below the navel. With one flat hand over the other, and both hands at a slight angle, press in and lightly down. Find the pulsing aorta to the left of the tan tien point and the inferior vena cava on the right of the tan tien point.

2. Press lightly to break up sedimentation in the aorta and vena cava. At the same time, feel for any blockages or tangles. Release blockages with longer finger pressure or small finger circles over the restriction.

3. Work your way down the lower abdomen a few centimeters at a time, repeating step 2 until you reach the pubic bone.

4. Work in the same way from the solar plexus down to the navel.

KARSAI NEI TSANG

⚙ Releasing the Energy Meridians: Karsai I and II
(Pages 44–45)

1. With your right hand over your left, press your fingers into the abdomen below the navel. Push in and slightly downward—toward the pubic bone.
2. Hold the pressure until you feel a release—a softening, a return of energy, or a warming sensation.
3. Move your hands down a few centimeters and repeat, working your way down to the pubic bone.

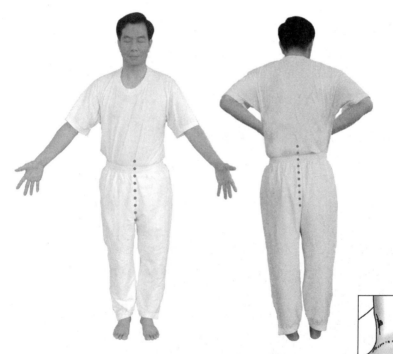

Karsai I and II energy meridians

Releasing the Karsai I and II energy meridians

❋ Releasing the Energy Meridians: Karsai III and IV

(Pages 46–47)

1. With your left hand over your right, press your hands into the abdomen below the navel. Push in and pull lightly downward at a 45-degree angle—toward the midline of the inguinal ligament.
2. Hold the pressure until you feel a release.
3. Move your hands a few centimeters down the left side of the abdomen toward the inguinal ligament and repeat. Continue until you have worked your way down to the inguinal ligament, then repeat these steps on the right side of the abdomen.

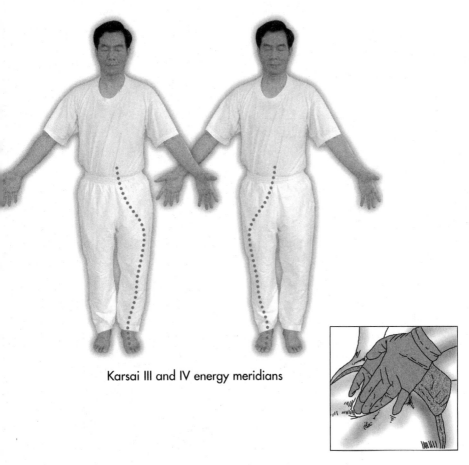

Karsai III and IV energy meridians

Releasing the Karsai III and IV energy meridians

☯ Massaging the Sexual Palace
(Page 51)

1. Place your two hands side by side with your fingers together, and press into the lower abdomen above the pubic bone.
2. Make small circular movements with the pads of your fingers, feeling for any congestion and knots. When you feel a restriction, pause and press with more intention, circling more directly into it. Ask your student to breathe into the restriction and release it upon exhalation.
3. Work from the right side over to the left side, from the area under the small intestine all the way down to the pubic bone.
4. When the superficial layer is released, repeat this sequence, gently moving your fingers deeper to access the tangles of the nerves and the deeper circulatory flow. The deeper you work the slower your movements should be.

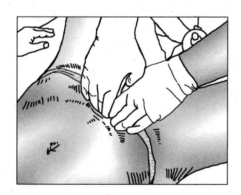

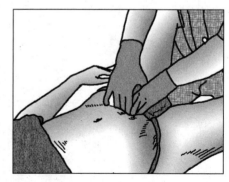

Massaging the Sexual Palace

Massage and Lymphatic Drainage over the Inguinal Ligament

(Pages 52–54)

1. Using the pads of your fingers or the outside of your thumb, press into the base of the inguinal ligament where it attaches at the pubic bone.
2. Slowly move up along the ligament—feeling it lengthen—until you reach its attachment at the crest of the pelvis.
3. Repeat this movement a few times until you feel the ligament soften and relax.
4. Place the flat of your fingers over the inguinal ligaments, working both sides at the same time. Make gentle pushing movements toward the navel.
5. Feel the lymphatic ducts releasing and the lymphatic fluid flushing to the deeper nodes.
6. Repeat several times on both sides.

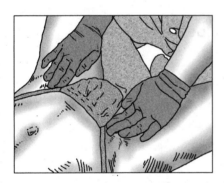
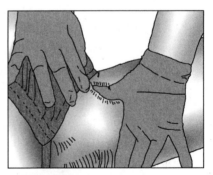
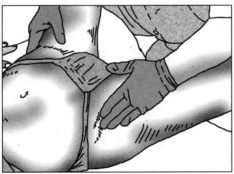

Releasing the inguinal ligament and lymphatic flow

KARSAI NEI TSANG (FEMALE)

Do not work on women during their menstruation, women using an IUD, women who are pregnant, or women with venereal disease or cancer.

🌀 Opening and Releasing the Uterus
(Pages 55–58)

1. Standing at your student's side, place your eight fingers to one side of the uterus and your thumbs together on the opposite side.
2. Press in with the flats of your fingers and pull the uterus toward your thumbs. Next, press in on your thumbs and push toward your fingers.
3. Continue kneading the uterus between your fingers and thumbs. Massage any tangles or twists.
4. Hold the uterus in the center for a while with both of your hands.
5. Stand on the other side of your student and repeat steps 1–4.

🌀 Releasing the Fallopian Tubes
(Pages 58–59)

1. With your fingers together, apply gentle circular massage over the fallopian tubes. Start at the uterus and work your way over to the ovary.
2. Notice if you feel any crimping or twisting in the tube—the fallopian tube and veins can become twisted. Slowly massage out any twists, knots, or tangles. Repeat on the other side.

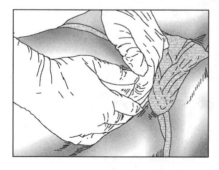

Opening and releasing the uterus

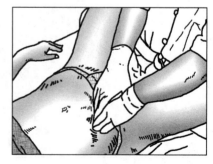

Releasing the fallopian tubes and ovaries

☯ Releasing the Ovaries
(Pages 59–61)

1. Touch the ovaries and feel their energy flow. Feel whether the two ovaries are properly aligned; they should be approximately even in height. Also check to feel if one ovary is closer to the skin surface than the other.
2. If one of the ovaries is not properly positioned, press into it with your fingers together, flat and relaxed.
3. Make small circular movements and free the ligamentous connections to the ovary. Then massage directly into the ovary and feel for the return of chi flow. Releasing congestion in the surrounding area can help the ovaries return to their proper place.
4. Repeat steps 2 and 3 on the other ovary.
5. Bring your awareness to the arteries and veins around the ovaries. It is possible that they have become tangled or knotted together with the ovaries. Patiently work out the tangles and knots with massage.

☯ Releasing the Urogenital Diaphragm
(Pages 61–65)

1. Bring your left hand over to the student's left labia majora and use the flat of your fingers to pull the labia over to the student's right side.
2. With your left hand stabilizing the genitals, use your right thumb to massage up the outside of the labium, along the ischiocavernosus muscle. When you feel knots, tangles, or congestion, press in and pull

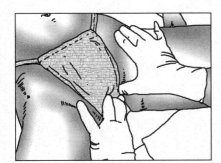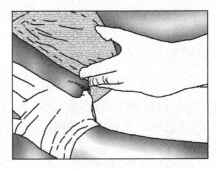

Releasing the urogenital diaphragm

the tissues toward the crease of the leg. Repeat this gentle pull many times, until you feel the area soften and the chi flow return.

3. If you feel a spiraling of the muscle or a tangling of the veins and nerves, work slowly to untangle them. Continue to repeat your gestures until you feel the area soften and the chi flow return.

4. Repeat steps 1–3 on the other side.

� Lifting the Uterus

(Pages 65–66)

1. Stand at your student's side, facing the pelvis. The student's knees should be up. Shape your hands like the bottom of a bowl and scoop up the underside of the uterus.

2. Lift the uterus gently but firmly upward toward the solar plexus. This will not be a perfectly linear movement; try to follow the body's path of least resistance.

3. After repeating these movements a few times, spread the sexual energy as in the exercise below.

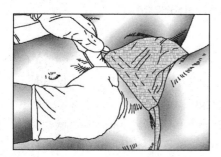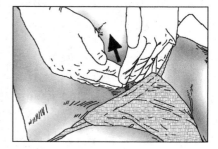

Lifting the uterus

� Lifting the Ovaries

(Pages 66–67)

1. Standing at the student's side, reach across to her opposite side and scoop into the inside rim of the pelvis with the flat surface of your eight fingers.

2. Gently lift the ovary and move it in a superior and medial direction,

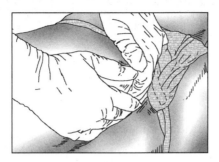

Lifting the Ovaries

stretching it up away from the pelvis and slightly toward the midline. Be sensitive to the direction the tissues move and follow the path of least resistance.

3. Move to the opposite side and repeat for the other ovary.

Spreading the Energy
(Page 67)

1. Sit between your student's lower legs, stretch out your right or left leg, and press the sole of your foot into her pelvic floor.
2. Hold the pressure for 2–3 minutes. Invite your student to feel the chi flowing in her body, whether it is flowing upward or downward.

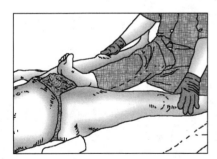 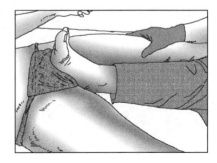

Spreading the Energy

KARSAI NEI TSANG (MALE)

Releasing Blood Supply to the Testicles and Penis
(Pages 79–80)

1. With your right hand, lift the testicles and penis and stabilize them up and over toward the student's left side.
2. Place your left thumb on the lower right edge of the right scrotal sac. Move your thumb upward, following the edge of the scrotal sac and the crease of the leg.
3. When you feel a deposit, in the veins, work this area with a small circular movement, pressing into the restriction. When the restriction eases, continue to move upward along the edge of the scrotal sac.
4. Repeat steps 1–3 on the student's left side. Finish by smoothing out the area with long, lighter strokes.

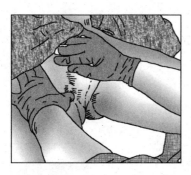

Releasing the blood supply to the genitals

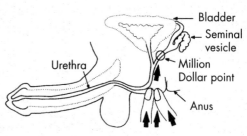

The Million Dollar point

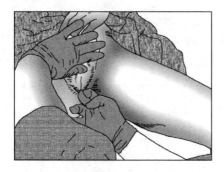

Energizing the prostate through the perineum: supine position

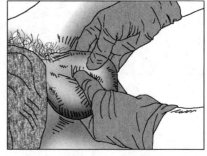

Releasing sedimentation in the scrotal sac

Energizing the Prostate through the Perineum: Supine Position

(Pages 80–81)

1. With your left hand, lift the testicles and penis upward and stabilize them away from the perineum.
2. With the pad of your right middle finger, push directly into the Million Dollar point—just in front of the anus and behind the perineum—until you feel the base of the prostate. Hold this pressure until you feel the prostate vitalized with chi.

Releasing Sedimentation in the Scrotal Sac

(Pages 81–83)

This technique should be used only on the superior boundary of the testicles. Do not work on the sides of the testicles or the inferior border of the testicles. This can cause serious problems.

1. Sitting between the student's legs, place your eight fingers under the testicles and let the weight of the testicles rest in your hands.
2. Place your left thumb between the two testicles, stabilizing the left testicle by pressing your left thumb down to meet your left fingers.
3. Press down with your right thumb into the superior boundary of the right testicle, holding the underside of the testicle firmly with your fingers. With your right thumb and fingers, search the veins just above the testicle for sedimentation or sand in the veins.
4. Press into the sediment with small circular movements until you feel it dissolve between your fingers and thumb.
5. Continue working the sandy areas one by one, then repeat steps 1–5 for the left testicle.

⟳ Improving Circulation in the Scrotal Sac

(Pages 83–85)

1. Place your fingers under the scrotal sac—supporting the testicles—and place your thumbs on top of the scrotal sac, superior to the testicles.
2. Gently move your thumbs along the veins in the scrotal sac to the base of the penis.
3. Repeat this movement a few times, balancing and smoothing out the chi flow.
4. Press your middle finger into the top of the scrotal sac toward the side and base of the penis. Sweep your finger from side to side, stimulating the circulation of the testicles and penis. If you find a restriction, pause and press into it while you make small circular movements.

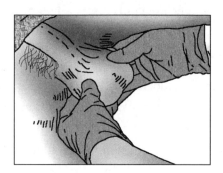

Smoothing out the veins in the
upper scrotal sac

⟳ Testicle Palm Rub

(Pages 85–86)

1. Firmly wrap your left thumb and forefinger around the base of the scrotal sac and slightly rotate the testicles clockwise to the right. This will place the testicles under a bit of tension in a small space at the bottom of the scrotal sac.
2. With the palm of your right hand, rub in a circular motion, somewhat vigorously, all around the sides and base of the testicles.
3. Now use your right thumb and forefinger to encircle the base of the

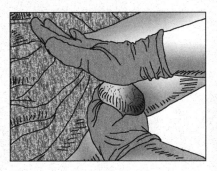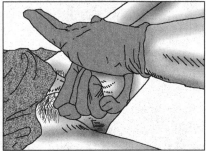

Testicle rub

scrotum and rotate the testicles counterclockwise to the left. Use your left palm to massage the testicles as described in step 2.

Energizing the Prostate through the Perineum on All Fours

(Page 94)

1. With your student kneeling on all fours, stabilize the sacrum with your left hand and press your right thumb or middle finger directly into the Million Dollar point, which is just in front of the anus and behind the perineum.
2. Press in firmly until you feel you are in contact with the prostate, then feel for any congestion.
3. Release your pressure when you feel the prostate release and flow with energy.

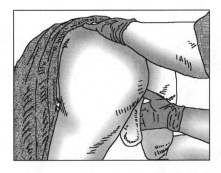

Energizing the prostate through the
perineum on all fours

Releasing the Inner Thigh

(Page 87)

1. With your student lying on his back, rotate the right leg exteriorly to expose the inside of the right leg. In this position the gracilis and adductor muscles will contract and bulge out a bit.
2. Place your right hand over the genitals. On men, stabilize the genitals toward the student's left side.
3. Place your left thumb underneath the bulging muscles and press toward the outer edge of the body.
4. Massage with a long stroke down the inside of the leg, repeating the stroke until you feel the leg release and the muscles soften.

The following techniques are performed with the student prone on all fours, resting his weight on his knees and his elbows. The practitioner sits on the table facing the student's pelvis.

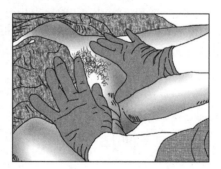

Releasing the inner thigh

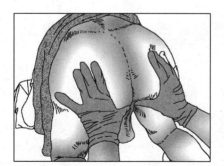
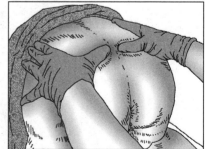

Releasing the buttocks and sacrum

⚛ Massaging the Buttocks and Sacrum
(Pages 88–89)

1. Place both hands flat on the student's buttocks, with your thumbs at the level of the ischial tuberosities and your fingers out to the sides of the buttocks.
2. Move your thumbs upward along the edges of the sacrum, feeling for restrictions as you go. When you feel a blockage, pause and press in on it, making small circular movements as needed.
3. As you reach the tip of the pelvic crest, bring your fingers and thumbs together, then sweep your hands down along the outsides of the pelvis.
4. Repeat steps 2 and 3 a few times, continuing to work on any restrictions you find.

⚛ Releasing and Balancing the Anococcygeal Region
(Pages 90–92)

1. Between the anus and the coccyx: Stabilize the right crest of the pelvis with your right hand. With your left thumb, press into the left side of the anococcygeal ligament, between the coccyx and anus. Press in on any restrictions until you feel a return of chi flow.
2. Move your thumb directly under the coccyx and above the anus, and press again into the anococcygeal ligament. Press into any twisting or stagnation in the ligament.
3. Now move your right thumb just to the right of the ligament and press in until you feel a return of chi flow.

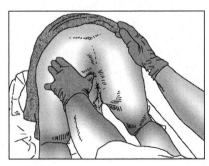

Releasing the anococcygeal ligament

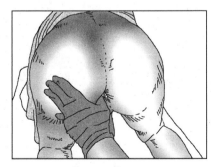

Releasing the anus

4. Releasing the anus: Stabilize the pelvis by placing your right hand on the right pelvic crest. Place your left thumb near the left side of the anus and the rest of your hand around the left buttock. Press in with your thumb and pull slightly to the left. Feel this space open and relax. Repeat for the other side.

Releasing Sciatic Nerve on All Fours
(Pages 92–93)

1. Press your thumbs into the pathway of the sciatic nerve. Feel for any knots and tangles and make small circular movements to release the restrictions.

Forearm Press—Anus to Sacrum
(Page 93)

The following technique is performed with the student prone and the practitioner kneeling on the table facing the student's pelvis.

1. Lean over the student's buttocks and place your forearm, ulna side down, along the midline from the anus to the sacrum.
2. Allow your body weight to sink into your forearm for 2–3 minutes, and feel your student's energy flow up the spine.

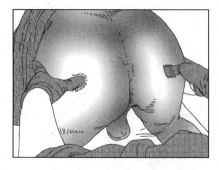

Releasing the sciatic nerve

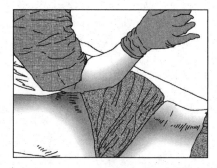

Forearm press—anus to sacrum

⟳ Massaging the Abdomen and Inguinal Ligament from Underneath

(Pages 96–97)

1. With your student on all fours, stand to his right side, with your right side touching the massage table.

2. Place your right hand over the lumbar vertebrae while the finger pads of your left hand scoop under the lower ribs and massage down the ascending colon and down to the pubic bone.

3. Repeat this sweeping motion a few times, then move to the opposite side and repeat for the descending colon and across to the sigmoid colon.

4. Standing on the student's right side again, place your left hand around the outside of his right thigh. With the finger pads of your right hand, massage down the length of the inguinal ligament. Repeat this movement a few times and then treat the other side.

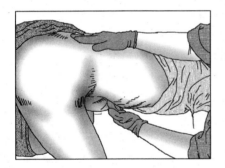
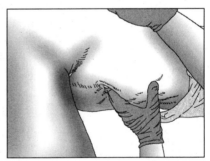
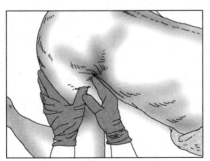

Massaging the abdomen and inguinal ligament from underneath

KARSAI NEI TSANG

☯ Herbal Packs for Women and Men
(Pages 76–77 and 97–99)

1. Press the herbal ball into the upper abdomen and make fairly rapid circular motions on the skin. Use the whole ball—the bottom and all the sides—to rotate the herbs over the skin.

2. Work your way down to the pubic bone, being careful to reach to the sides of the abdomen.

3. Spend extra time with the herbal ball in the lower abdomen, where so much of the massage took place.

4. Ask your student if the herbal ball is too hot before pressing it directly on the genitals. For men, move the penis away from the testicles; then place the herbal ball on the upper side of the testicles.

5. When the herbal ball is at a good temperature, press it into the vulva or the upper side of the testicles and hold for 15 seconds or so. Move the herbal ball to each side of the testicles, pressing and holding for about 15 seconds each time.

6. Finish the massage by moving the herbal ball to the posterior pelvic floor for women or the base of the testicles for men. Feel the energy move up through the central channel to the pineal gland.

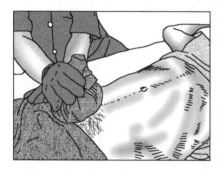 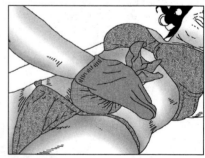

Herbal packs

TAI CHI WU STYLE
The Three-Direction Short Wu Form

⟳ Opening Movements

(Pages 109–12)

1. Beginning stance: Stand facing north, with your feet relaxed and together. Feel your head suspended from a string connected to the heavenly force.
2. Smile down to your navel, then inhale, round the scapulae, sink the chest, and open the armpits. Exhale and sink down. Shift tailbone to your right heel as you lift the left heel.

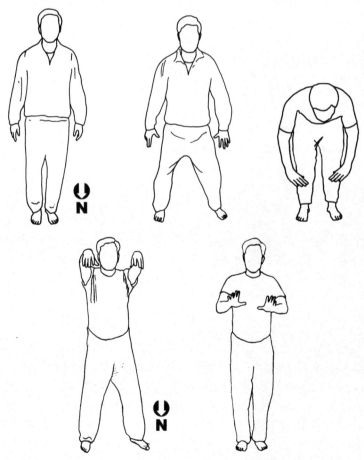

Opening the form

3. Inhale and pick up the left foot, then exhale and set down the left foot a shoulder's width apart from the right foot. Stand in Iron Shirt posture.

4. Lower your upper body from the hips and drop your head down. Raise your upper body and arms from the wrists. Lower your hands.

Core Movements First Round: Right-Hand Form Facing North

(Pages 112–21)

1. Bird's Tail/Ward Off Strike: Shift tailbone to right heel–draw out and hook left foot forming ball with hands–Ward Off to the north.

2. Bird's Tail/Rollback: Slip left fingers to right wrist forming circle to the east–shift tailbone to left heel and lift up right heel opening the hip to the east.

3. Bird's Tail/Press: Lift right foot and place the right heel down–place left fingers on right wrist and Press forward to the east–Rollback, sinking back on left heel.

4. Bird's Tail/Strike: Pull back the right palm and Push forward to the east, shifting tailbone to right heel.

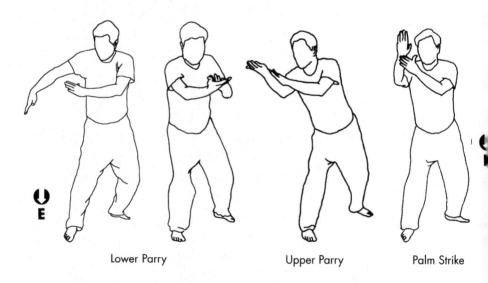

Lower Parry   Upper Parry   Palm Strike

Right-Hand Form (to north): Bird's Tail and Palm Strike

5. Single Whip: Form beak with right hand to the southeast–step left foot back–draw right palm across with eyes following–strike out to the northwest with palm.

6. Flying Oblique: Raise left palm–circle right hand down, crossing at midsection–shift tailbone to right heel.

7. Lift Hand Step Forward: Raise right hand above head–bring left hand to knee.

8. White Crane Spreads Its Wings: Shift tailbone to left heel forming chi ball at midsection with both palms–draw right foot up–stand in Iron Shirt stance.

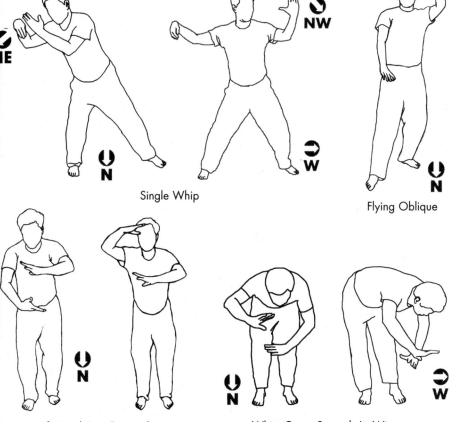

Single Whip

Flying Oblique

Lift Hand Step Forward

White Crane Spreads Its Wings

Right-Hand Form (to north): Single Whip, Flying Oblique, Lift Hand Step Forward, and White Crane Spreads Its Wings

9. Transition to Left-Hand Form: Lower upper body from hips–drop head–turn hips to left, circling a chi ball over the head to the right side–shift tailbone to right heel.

10. Brush Knee: Step left heel back to south–turn right foot 45 degrees west–drop left hand, brushing left knee–shift tailbone to center–push right hand forward.

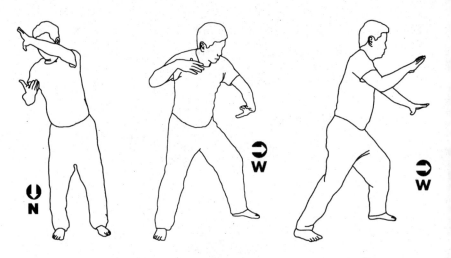

Right-Hand Form (to north): Brush Knee transitioning to
Left-Hand Form to west

⟳ Core Movements Second Round: Left-Hand Form Facing West

(Pages 121–29)

1. Bird's Tail/Ward Off: Shift tailbone to right heel–draw left fingers to right wrist–circle forward, shifting right fingers to left wrist, then circle back.

2. Bird's Tail/Press: Press right fingers forward on right wrist–move hips to west, then circle hips back to northwest for the Palm Strike.

3. Bird's Tail/Push: Lift back left fingers–push hips to west.

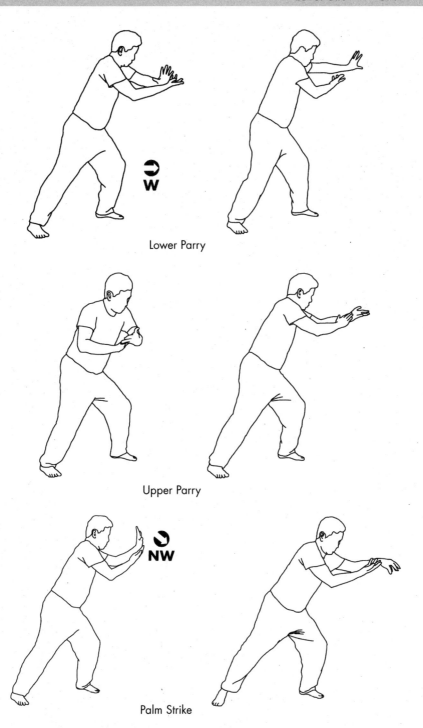

Lower Parry

Upper Parry

Palm Strike

Left-Hand Form (to west): Bird's Tail and Palm Strike

4. Single Whip: Form beak with left hand in northwest corner–step right foot back–draw right palm across with eyes following–strike out to the northeast with palm.

5. Flying Oblique: Raise right palm–circle left hand down, crossing at midsection–shift tailbone to left heel.

6. Lift Hand Step Forward: Raise right hand above head–bring left hand to knee.

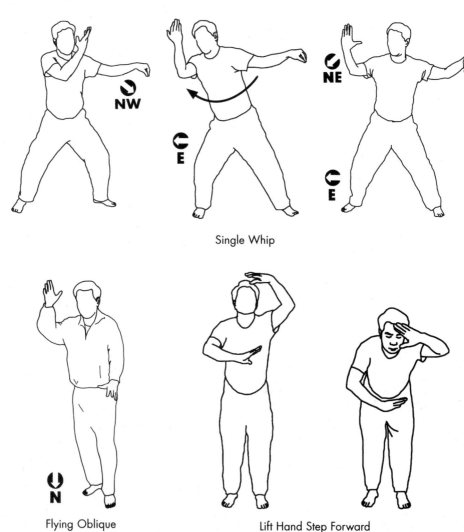

Single Whip

Flying Oblique   Lift Hand Step Forward

Left-Hand Form (to west): Single Whip, Flying Oblique,
Lift Hand Step Forward

7. White Crane: Shift tailbone to right heel, forming chi ball at midsection with both palms–draw left foot up into Iron Shirt stance.

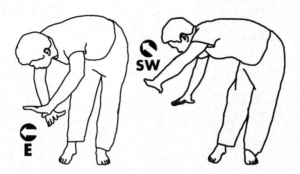

Left-Hand Form (to west): White Crane Spreads Its Wings

8. Transition to Right-Hand Form: Lower upper body from hips–drop head–turn hips to right, circling chi ball over head to left side–shift tailbone to left heel.

9. Brush Knee/Changing Directions (180°): Step back with right foot pointing south, opening hips to south–draw right hand down (crossing waist) to protect right knee–Press left hand south.

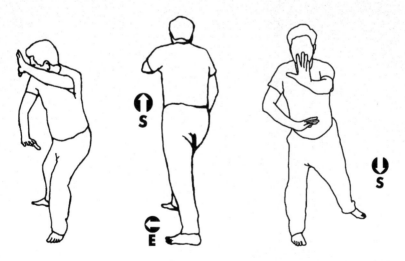

Left-Hand Form (to west): Brush Knee and transition
to Right-Hand Form facing south

🌀 Core Movements Third Round: Right-Hand Form Facing South

(Pages 130–39)

1. Bird's Tail/Ward Off: Shift tailbone to left heel–circle right hand back across left wrist–shift left fingers to right wrist and circle back.
2. Bird's Tail/Press: With left fingers Press right wrist forward–sink back–shift tailbone to left heel–right hand back.
3. Bird's Tail/Push: Move hips 2 counts forward—to the south.
4. Single Whip: Form beak with right hand in the southeast corner–step left foot back, drawing left palm across with eyes following–strike out with palm to the northeast.
5. Flying Oblique to east: Raise left palm–circle down right hand crossing at midsection–shift tailbone to right heel.
6. Lift Hand Step Forward: Raise left hand above head–bring right hand to knee.
7. White Crane Spreads Its Wings: Shift tailbone to left heel while forming chi ball at midsection with both palms–draw right foot up into Iron Shirt stance.

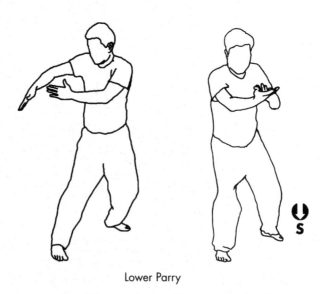

Lower Parry

Right-Hand Form facing south: Bird's Tail (Lower Parry)

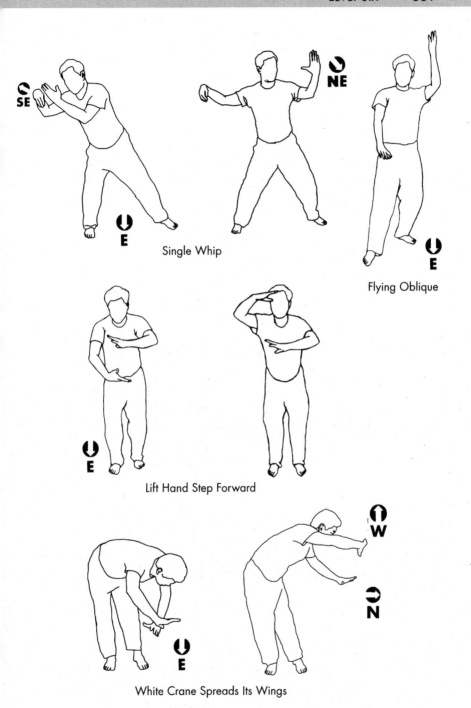

Single Whip

Flying Oblique

Lift Hand Step Forward

White Crane Spreads Its Wings

Right-Hand Form facing south: Single Whip, Flying Oblique, Lift Hand Step Forward, White Crane Spreads Its Wings

8. Transition to Left-Hand Form: Lower upper body from hips–drop head–turn hips to left, circling chi ball over the head to the right side–shift tailbone to right heel.

9. Brush Knee: Step left heel back to south–turn right foot 45 degrees west–drop left hand brushing left knee–shift tailbone to center–push right hand forward.

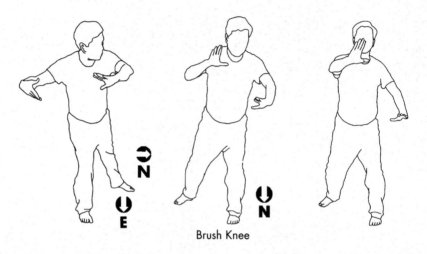

Brush Knee

Right-Hand Form facing south: Brush Knee

TAI CHI WU STYLE
The Eight-Direction Short Wu Form

⬯ Core Movements Rounds 4–7 (SW, NE, NW, SE Corners) and Completion

(Pages 140–46)

1. Fourth round, SE Corner, Left-Hand Form: Bird's Tail to north–Single Whip to southeast–Flying Oblique, Lift Hand Step Forward, and White Crane facing east–Brush Knee strike to southeast–change directions 180°.

2. Fifth round, NW Corner, Right-Hand Form: Bird's Tail to southeast–Single Whip to northeast–Flying Oblique, Lift Hand Step Forward, and White Crane facing east–Brush Knee strike to northwest–change directions 135°.

3. Sixth round, SW Corner, Left-Hand Form: Bird's Tail to northwest–Single Whip to northeast–Flying Oblique, Lift Hand Step Forward, and White Crane facing north–Brush Knee strike to southwest–change directions 180°.

4. Seventh round, NE Corner, Right-Hand Form: Bird's Tail strike to southwest–Single Whip to southeast–Flying Oblique, Lift Hand Step Forward, and White Crane facing south–Brush Knee strike to northeast–change directions 45°.

⬯ Closing the Form

5. Completion: Shift tailbone to right hip and release transition. Open both hands, moving them up, outward, and downward. Draw left foot straight back, setting it down next to the right foot. Shift tailbone to the left heel and lift up the right leg, placing it parallel with the left. Draw feet together with toes even.

6. Cross Hands: Raise hands 12 inches in front of body to form an X below the shoulders, with the left hand closer to the body.

7. Distribute weight evenly between both feet. Simultaneously straighten body and lower hands to sides with palms facing back. End all movements at the same time.

8. Relax and center yourself; feel the chi expand in your body. Collect energy at your navel.

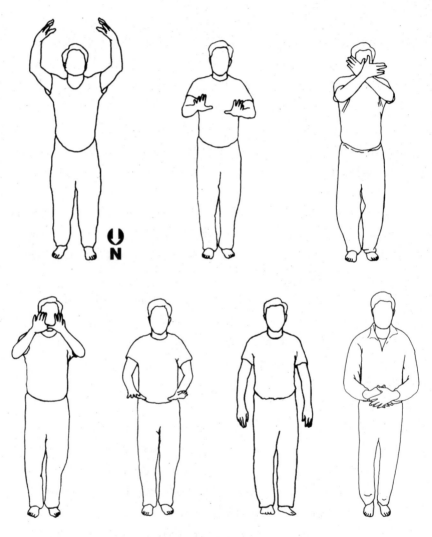

Closing the Form

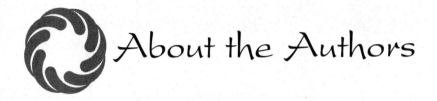

About the Authors

MANTAK CHIA

Mantak Chia has been studying the Taoist approach to life since childhood. His mastery of this ancient knowledge, enhanced by his study of other disciplines, has resulted in the development of the Universal Healing Tao system, which is now being taught throughout the world.

Mantak Chia was born in Thailand to Chinese parents in 1944. When he was six years old, he learned from Buddhist monks how to sit and "still the mind." While in grammar school he learned traditional Thai boxing, and he soon went on to acquire considerable skill in aikido, yoga, and Tai Chi. His studies of the Taoist way of life began in earnest when he was a student in Hong Kong, ultimately leading to his mastery of a wide variety of esoteric disciplines, with the guidance of several masters, including Master I Yun, Master Meugi, Master Cheng Yao Lun, and Master Pan Yu. To better understand the mechanisms behind healing energy, he also studied Western anatomy and medical sciences.

Master Chia has taught his system of healing and energizing practices to tens of thousands of students and trained more than two thousand instructors and practitioners throughout the world. He has established centers for Taoist study and training in many countries around the globe. In June of 1990, he was honored by the International Congress of Chinese Medicine and Qi Gong (Chi Kung), which named him the Qi Gong Master of the Year.

WILLIAM U. WEI

Born after World War II, growing up in the Midwest area of the United States, and trained in Catholicism, William Wei became a student of the Tao started studying under Master Mantak Chia in the early 1980s. In the later 1980s he became a senior instructor of the Universal Healing Tao, specializing in one-on-one training. In the early 1990s William Wei moved to Tao Garden, Thailand, and assisted Master Mantak Chia in building Tao Garden Taoist Training Center. For six years William traveled to over thirty countries, teaching with Master Mantak Chia and serving as marketing and construction coordinator for the Tao Garden. Upon completion of Tao Garden in December 2000, he became project manager for all the Universal Tao publications and products. With the purchase of a mountain with four waterfalls in southern Oregon, USA, in the late 1990s, William Wei is presently completing a Taoist Mountain Sanctuary for personal cultivation, higher-level practices, and ascension. William Wei is the coauthor with Master Chia of *Sexual Reflexology, Living in the Tao,* and the Taoist poetry book of 366 daily poems, *Emerald River,* which expresses the feeling, essence, and stillness of the Tao. He is also the cocreator with Master Mantak Chia of the Universal Healing Tao Chi Cards, upon which this book has been based, under the pen name "The Professor—Master of Nothingness, the Myth that takes the Mystery out of Mysticism." William U. Wei, also known as Wei Tzu, is a pen name for this instructor so the instructor can remain anonymous and can continue to become a blade of grass in a field of grass.

The Universal
Healing Tao
System and
Training Center

THE UNIVERSAL HEALING TAO SYSTEM

The ultimate goal of Taoist practice is to transcend physical boundaries through the development of the soul and the spirit within the human. That is also the guiding principle behind the Universal Healing Tao, a practical system of self-development that enables individuals to complete the harmonious evolution of their physical, mental, and spiritual bodies. Through a series of ancient Chinese meditative and internal energy exercises, the practitioner learns to increase physical energy, release tension, improve health, practice self-defense, and gain the ability to heal him- or herself and others. In the process of creating a solid foundation of health and well-being in the physical body, the practitioner also creates the basis for developing his or her spiritual potential by learning to tap into the natural energies of the sun, moon, earth, stars, and other environmental forces.

The Universal Healing Tao practices are derived from ancient techniques rooted in the processes of nature. They have been gathered and integrated into a coherent, accessible system for well-being that works directly with the life force, or chi, that flows through the meridian system of the body.

Master Chia has spent years developing and perfecting techniques for teaching these traditional practices to students around the world through ongoing classes, workshops, private instruction, and healing sessions, as well as books and video and audio products. Further information can be obtained at www.universal-tao.com.

THE UNIVERSAL HEALING TAO TRAINING CENTER

The Tao Garden Resort and Training Center in northern Thailand is the home of Master Chia and serves as the worldwide headquarters for Universal Healing Tao activities. This integrated wellness, holistic health, and training center is situated on eighty acres surrounded by the beautiful Himalayan foothills near the historic walled city of Chiang Mai. The serene setting includes flower and herb gardens ideal for meditation, open-air pavilions for practicing Chi Kung, and a health and fitness spa.

The center offers classes year round, as well as summer and winter retreats. It can accommodate two hundred students, and group leasing can be arranged. For information on courses, books, products, and other resources, see below.

RESOURCES

Universal Healing Tao Center
274 Moo 7, Luang Nua, Doi Saket, Chiang Mai, 50220 Thailand
Tel: (66)(53) 495-596 Fax: (66)(53) 495-852
E-mail: universaltao@universal-tao.com
Web site: www.universal-tao.com

For information on retreats and the health spa, contact:
Tao Garden Health Spa & Resort
E-mail: info@tao-garden.com, taogarden@hotmail.com
Web site: www.tao-garden.com

Good Chi • Good Heart • Good Intention

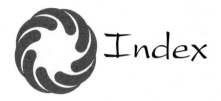

Index

Page numbers in *italics* refer to illustrations.

abdomen, 291–92, *291*, 371
Absorbing the Earth Force, 139
Absorbing the Heavenly Force,
   138–39, *138*
Activating the Three Fires, 202, *202*
Advanced Chi Nei Tsang, 271
   Abdomen, 291–92, *291*
   Applications for Specific Ailments,
      299–301, *299–301*
   Chest, 295
   Heart, 294, *294*
   Heat and Cold, 298
   Kidneys, 288–89, *288*
   Legs and Feet, 295
   Liver, Pericardium, Heart, 286–87,
      286
   Muscle Cramps, 292–93, *292–93*
   Nerves and Back, 296–98, *297*
   Opening the Wind Gates at the
      Navel, 284–85, *285*
   Pain, Numbness, and Heat, 296
   Tongue, Eyes, and Head, 287
   Vena Cava, Aorta, and Lumbar
      Plexus, 289–90, *289–90*

affirmations, 205–7
Alchemy of Sexual Energy, 12, 24–29,
   25–26, 28–29
Alcor, 349
Alioth, 349
anger, 300
Animal Postures, 230–35, *230–35*
Animal Protection Practice, 352–53,
   353
anococcygeal region, 369–70, *369*
aorta, 289–90
Aquarius, 247–48
Aries, 247–48
arthritis, 301
as above, so below, 1
astrology, 247–48
auras, 152–53, 266–67, *267*

back, 296–98
Back Line, 17–18, *17*
Balanced Bow, 219, *219*
balancing chi, 3–4
Balancing the Planetary and Stellar
   Influences, 280–81, *280*

Balancing Yin/Yang Extremes in the
Star World, 281–82, *282*
Balancing Your Inner Climate,
100–102, *100*
Bamboo Swinging in the Wind, 226,
226
Bear posture, 231, *231*
Belt Channels, 196–98, *196*
Big Dipper, 347–48, *348*
bioelectromagnetism, 1
Bird's Tail, 320
Birth of the Immortal Fetus, 106
black, 332
black holes, *282*
black turtle, 352
bladder, 343
blood vessels, 330
blue light, 349
Boar, 248
Bone Breathing, 79–80, *79*
Bone Compression, 81–82, *81*
Bone Marrow Nei Kung, 70–71
Bone Compression, 81–82, *81*
Female Chi Weight Lifting, 96–97, *97*
Female Sexual Energy Massage,
91–93, *91, 93*
Male Chi Weight Lifting, 94–95, *95*
Male Sexual Energy Massage, 88–90,
89
Rattan Stick Hitting, 78
Scrotal Compression, 85
Sexual Power Lock Practice (male),
86–87, *86*
Testicle Breathing, 83–85, *84*
Wire Rod Hitting, 73–78, *74, 77*
Bones, 28–29, *28–29*

bouncing, 236
Bright Yang, 349
Buddha Palm Closing Practices, 140–
42, *141*
Buddha Palm Opening Practices, 136–
39, *137–38*
Buffalo, 248
Bull posture, 235, *235*
Butterfly Protection, 263–66, *265*
buttocks, 369

Cancer, 247–48
Capricorn, 247–48
Cellular Cleansing, 242
cerebellum, 349
Channeling the Earth Force, 136–38
Chasing the Winds, 157
Chen, 183, 186
chest, 295
chi, 1, 3–5
Chia, Mantak, 2, 385
Chien, 184, 186
Chi Nei Tsang, 2–3, 133
Balancing the Pulses, 173
Detoxifying the Organs, 164–70,
164, 166–67, 169–70
Detoxifying the Skin and the Large
and Small Intestines, 160–63, *161*
Fanning Hot Sick Energy, 154, *154,
154–55*
Healing Hands Meditation, 152–53,
153
Navel Diagnosis and Release,
158–59, *158–59*
Opening the Wind Gates, 156–57,
156

Releasing Knots, Tangles, and
   Nerves, 163
Releasing Toxins from the Lymph
   System, 171–73, *171–72*
Treating Common Ailments,
   176–78, *177–78*
Tree Chi Kung, 179–81, *179, 181*
Venting Hot Sick Energy, 155, *155*
Working on the Sexual Organs,
   174–75, *174–75*
Chinese animals, 248
Ching Chi, 333
Chi Self-Massage, 13–14, 34–39, *34,*
   37–38
chlorophyll liquid concentrate, 244
cinnabar, 333
Circle of Fire, 203
coffee, 244
cold, 298
Collect Energy in the Navel, 19, *19*
Colonic System, 243–44, *243*
common ailments, 176–78, *177–78*
compassion fire, 333
Connecting Heaven and Earth,
   143–44, *143*
Connecting the Senses, 102–3
Connecting to the Stellar and Galactic
   Forces, 278–79, *279*
Connecting with the Big Dipper,
   347–48, *348*
conserving chi, 3
Cosmic Astrology, 212, 247–48
Cosmic Detox, 211, 242–46, *242–46*
Cosmic Fusion, 133–34
   Advanced Practice Formulas,
      199–201, *199, 201*

Creation Cycle, 187–89, *187, 189*
   Forming the Pakuas, 182–86, *182,*
      185
   Opening the Belt Channels, 196–98,
      196
   Opening the Thrusting Channels,
      190–95, *191, 195*
Cosmic Healing, 2–3, 4, 270
Cosmic Orbit Meditation, 26–29, *26,*
      28–29
Coupling, 334–36, *335*
courage, 333
Crane posture, 231, *231*
Crane's Beak, 142
cranial nerves, 349
Creation Cycle, 187–89, *187, 189*
Cricket Rests on Flower, 220
Crocodile Lifts Head, 217–18, *217*
crown, 193
Cutting from the Third Eye, 263–64
Cutting the Senses, 264, *265*

Destructive Army, 349
Detoxifying the Organs, 164–70, *164,*
      166–70, 169–70
Detoxifying the Skin and the Large
   and Small Intestines, 160–63, *161*
diaphragm, 164–65, *164*, 190, 192
digestive tract, 17, *17*
Dog, 248
Door of Life, 27, 240–41, *241*, 352
Dragon, 248
Dragon Gazes at the Pearl, 302–4,
   302–4
Dragon posture, 232, *232*
Drilling into the Head, 264, *265*

Dry Skin Brushing, 245–46, *245*

Dual Cultivation, 66–67, *67*

Dubhe, 349

Eagle posture, 232, *232*

Ears, Mouth, Face, 36–37, *37*

Earth, 212

Earth-Sun-Moon Triangle, 274–75, *274*

East and South Corners, Right-Hand Form, 130–31, *131*

Egg Exercise, 65, *65*

Eight-Direction Short Wu Form, 383–84, *383–84*

Eight Hand and Arm Positions, 250–53, *250–53*

Eighth Wind, 295

Elephant posture, 233

Eleventh Wind, 296–98

Embracing the Tree, 46, *47*

emotions, 104–5, *104*

Empty Force Breath, 227–28, *227*

Empty Force Exercises, 228–29, *229*

endocrine glands, 337, *337*

Energizing the Prostate through the Perineum, 365, 367

energy, learning to feel, 8

Energy Balance through the Tao, 208–9

Growing the Tendons, 223–26, *223–26*

Mind-Eye-Heart Power, 223–26, *223–26*

Spine, Psoas, and Ring Muscles, 215–22, *215–22*

Energy Body, 199–200, 268–69, *269*

energy protection formulas, 262–67, *262, 265, 267*

epsom salts, 244

expanding chi, 4

Eyes, 34–35, *35*

eyes, 287

facial pakua, 185–86, *185*

Fair Lady Jumps, 317, *317*

fairness, 333

fallopian tubes, 360

Fanning Hot Sick Energy, 154, *154*

feet, 39, 295

Female Chi Weight Lifting, 96–97, *97*

Female Sexual Energy Massage, 91–93, *91, 93*

Fifth Healing Sound, 44, *45*

Fifth Level, 5

Advanced Chi Nei Tsang, 271, 284–301, *285–86, 288–94, 297*

Golden Elixir Chi Kung, 272, 302–18, *302–6, 308–10, 312–18*

Tai Chi Fa Jin, 272–73, 319–27, *319–21, 323–25, 327*

Taoist Astral Healing, 270–71, 274–83, *274, 276, 279–80, 282–83*

Fifth Wind, 291–92, *291*

fingers, 140–42

Fire, 212

First Corner, South (Left-Hand Form), 320–21, *320–21*

First Healing Sound, 40–41, *40*

First Level

Healing Love Through the Tao, 59, *61, 62, 64–65, 67, 69*

Inner Smile, 10, 16–19, *16–19*

Iron Shirt Chi Kung, 14–15, 46–57, *47, 50, 52, 55*

Six Healing Sounds, 10–11, 40–45, *40, 42, 45*

Wisdom Chi Kung, 11–12, 20–23, *20–23*

First Wind, 286–87, *286*

Five Organs, Steaming, 336

foot and hand kicking, 236

Forearm Press, 370, *370*

Forming the Energy Body, 268–69, *269*

Four Pakuas, 98–99, *98*

Fourth Healing Sound, 43

Fourth Level, 5

　Cosmic Astrology, 247–48

　Cosmic Detox, 242–46, *242–46*

　Energy Balance Through the Tao, 208–9, 215–26, *215–26*

　Fusion of the Eight Psychic Channels, 258–69, *259–62, 265, 267, 269*

　Simple Chi Kung, 236–41, *237–39, 241*

　Tendon Nei Kung, 249–57, *250–55*

Fourth Wind, 289–90, *289–90*

Front Line, 16. *See also* Functional Channel

Full-Body Breathing, 215–17, *215–16*

Functional Channel, 13, 16, 147–49, *147–48*

Fusion of the Eight Psychic Channels, 213–14

　Butterfly Protection, 264–66, *265*

　Cutting from the Third Eye, 263–64

　Cutting the Senses, 264, *265*

Drilling into the Head, 264, *265*

Forming the Energy Body, 268–69, *269*

Opening the Great Bridge and Regulator Channels, 258–61, *258–61*

Sealing the Aura, 266–67, *267*

Spinal Cord Cutting, 262, *262*

Spinal Cord Microcosmic Orbit, 263

Fusion of the Five Elements, 71–72

　Advanced Fusion Practices, 106–12, *107, 111*

　Balancing Your Inner Climate, 100–102, *100*

　Birth of the Immortal Fetus, 106

　Connecting the Senses, 102–3

　Forming Four Pakuas and the Pearl, 98–99, *98*

　Transforming Emotions, 104–5, *104*

gallbladder, 345

Gall Bladder meridian, 345, *345*

garlic, 244

Gathering the Golden Earth Pill, 313–14, *313–14*

Gathering the Small Pill, 352–53, *353*

Gemini, 247–48

gentleness, 333

Giant Raises the Tower, 307–9, *308–9*

glycothymoline, 244

Golden Earth Pill, 313–14, *313–14*

Golden Elixir Chi Kung, 272

　Dragon Gazes at the Pearl, 302–4, *302–4*

　Ending Exercise, 318, *318*

Fair Lady Jumps, 317, *317*

Gathering the Golden Earth Pill, 313–14, *313–14*

Giant Raises the Tower, 307–9, *308–9*

Iron Bridge Swallow, 310–11, *310*

Iron Buffalo Plows the Land, 316–17, *316*

Looking Back at the Moon, 305, *305*

Pull the Silk and Swing the Leg, 311–12, *312*

Shaking the Head and Wagging the Tail, *310*, 311

Tiger Out of the Cage, 315–16, *315*

Wai T'o Offering the Rod, 305, *305*

Golden Phoenix Washes Its Feathers, 54–56, *55*

Golden Turtle Immersing in Water, 52–53, *52*

Governing Vessel, 28–29

Governor Channel, 13, 17–18, *17*

Grasping the Moon, 143–44, *143*

green dragon, 332, 352

Hand and Wrist Stretches, 239–40, *239*

Hands, Feet, Organs, and Glands, 38–39, *38*

happiness, 333

head, 287

headaches, 176

Healing Energy of Shared Consciousness, 134–35

Activating the Three Fires, 202, *202*

Circle of Fire, 203

Virtuous Mind Power, 205–7, *205–6*

World Link of Protection, 203–4, *204*

Healing Hands Meditation, 152–53, *153*

Healing Light of the Tao, 12–13, 30–33, *31–33*

Healing Love through the Tao, 15, 58–69, *59, 61, 62, 64–65, 67, 69*

heart, 39, 170, *170*, 286–87, 294, *294*, 300, 342

heart attacks, 299–300, *299*

heartbeat, 250

Heart Compassion Fire, 333

Heart Exercise, 43

Heart meridian, 342, *342*

Heart Protector, 170, *170*

heat, 296, 298

Heavenly Guard, 349

Herbal Packs, 371, *371*

hiatal hernia, 301, *301*

hip rotations, 236

Holding the Golden Urn, 50–51, *50*

Honest Chastity, 349

Horse, 248

Horse posture, 234, *234*

hot sick energy, 154–55, *154–55*

Huge Gate, 349

Hungry Wolf, 349

hypothalamus, 349

Immortal Tao, 2, 3, 6

Imperial Fire, 21

Implants, 244

Improving Circulation in the Scrotal Sac, 365
increasing chi, 4
Increasing the Pulse, 346, *346*
inguinal ligament, 359, 371
Inner Alchemy, 2
Inner Eye, 347
Inner Smile, 4, 10, 16–19, *16–19*
Inner Structure of Tai Chi, 72
    East and South Corners,
       Right-Hand Form, 130–31, *131*
    North Corner, Left-Hand Form,
       113–20, *114–15, 117–19*
    North Corner, Right-Hand Form,
       124–29, *124–29*
    Opening Movements, 113–16,
       114–15
    West, South, and North Corners,
       Transition to Right-Hand Form,
       120–23, *121–23*
inner thigh, 368
Intellectual Art, 349
Internal Alchemy, 133–34
intestines, 39
Iron Bar, 57
Iron Bridge, 56–57, *57*
Iron Bridge Swallow, 310–11, *310*
Iron Buffalo Plows the Land, 316–17,
    316
Iron Shirt Chi Kung, 14–15, 46–57,
    47, 50, 52, 55
Iron Shirt Packing Process, 46–49

jaw, 300
joy, 333
Jupiter, 352

Kan, 182, 185, 186, 328–29, 332–33,
    332. See also Taoist Soul Body
Karsai Ne Tsang, 329–30
    Female Practices, 360–63, *360–63*
    Herbal Packs, 371, *371*
    Male Practices, 364–71, *364,
       366–71*
    Massage and Lymphatic Drainage
       over the Inguinal Ligament, 359,
       359
    Massaging the Sexual Palace, 358,
       358
    Releasing the Energy Meridians,
       356–57
Ken, 184
Kidney Exercise, 41
Kidney meridian, 343, *343*
kidneys, 39, 169, *169*, 288–89, *288,
    343
kindness, 333
knee rotations, 236
knees, 39
knots, 163
Kun, 183–84, 186

Lady Shuttle, 320
large intestine, 160–62, 340–41
Large Intestine meridian, 340–41,
    340
lead, 332
legs, 295
lemon juice, 244
Leo, 247–48
Level Five, 5
    Advanced Chi Nei Tsang, 271,
       284–301, *285–86, 288–94, 297*

Golden Elixir Chi Kung, 272,
302–18, *302–6, 308–10, 312–18*
Tai Chi Fa Jin, 272–73, 319–27,
319–21, 323–25, 327
Taoist Astral Healing, 270–71,
274–83, *274, 276, 279–80,*
282–83
Level Four, 5
Cosmic Astrology, 247–48
Cosmic Detox, 242–46, *242–46*
Energy Balance Through the Tao,
208–9, 215–26, *215–26*
Fusion of the Eight Psychic
Channels, 258–69, *259–62, 265,*
267, 269
Simple Chi Kung, 236–41, *237–39,*
241
Tendon Nei Kung, 249–57, *250–55*
Level One, 5
Alchemy of Sexual Energy, 12,
24–29, *25–26, 28–29*
Chi Self-Massage, 13–14
goals of, 6–7
Healing Light of the Tao, 12–13,
30–33, *31–33*
Healing Love Through the Tao, 15,
58–69, *59, 61, 62, 64–65, 67, 69*
Inner Smile, 10, 16–19, *16–19*
Iron Shirt Chi Kung, 14–15, 46–57,
47, 50, 52, 55
Six Healing Sounds, 10–11, 40–45,
40, 42, 45
Wisdom Chi Kung, 11–12, 20–23,
20–23
Level Six, 5, 329–30
Karsai Ne Tsang, 354–72, *354,*

356–64, 366–71
Tai Chi Wu Style, 330–31
Taoist Soul Body, 328–29, 332–53,
332, 335–46, 353
Level Three, 5
Chi Nei Tsang, 133, 152–81, *153–56,*
158–59, 161, 164, 166–67,
169–72, 174–75, 177–79, 181
Cosmic Fusion, 133–34, 182–201,
182, 185, 187, 189, 191, 195–96,
199, 201
Healing Energy of Shared
Consciousness, 134–35, 202–7,
202, 204–6
Taoist Cosmic Healing, 132–33,
136–51, *137–38, 141, 143–45,*
147–48, 150
Level Two, 5
Bone Marrow Nei Kung, 70–71,
73–97, *74, 77, 81, 89, 91, 93, 95,*
97
Fusion of the Five Elements, 71–72,
98–112, *98, 100, 104, 107, 111*
Inner Structure of Tai Chi, 72,
113–31, *114–15, 117–19,*
121–29, 131
Li, 183, 185, 186, 328–29, *332. See*
also Taoist Soul Body
Libra, 247–48
Life and Death Point, 299–300, *299*
Lifting the Ovaries, 362–63, *362*
Lifting the Uterus, 362
Linking the Yang and Yin Arm Routes,
261
liver, 39, 167–68, *167*, 286–87, 300,
345

Liver Exercise, 42–43, *42*
Liver meridian, 345, *345*
Living Tao, 2
Looking Back at the Moon, 305
love, 333
Lower Abdominal Breathing, 46
lower back pain, 176–78, *177–78*
Lower Tan Tien, 27–28
lumbar plexus, 289–90
Lung Exercise, 40–41, *40*
Lung meridian, 340–41, *340*
lungs, 39, 165, 340–41
lymph system, 171–73, *171–72*,
    338–39

Male Chi Weight Lifting, 94–95, *95*
Male Sexual Energy Massage, 88–90,
    89
manifestations, 205–7
Marrow Washing, 136–39
Mars, 352
Martial Art, 349
massage
    Female Sexual Energy Massage,
        91–93, *91*, *93*
    Male Sexual Energy Massage, 88–90,
        89
Massaging the Abdomen and Inguinal
    Ligament, 371, *371*
Massaging the Buttocks and Sacrum,
    369
Megrez, 349
memory center, 349
Merak, 349
Mercury, 352
mercury, 333

Metal, 212
Microcosmic Orbit, 12, 30–33,
    31–33
Middle Line, 17, *17*
Middle Tan Tien, 27
Million Dollar point, *364*, 365
Ming Men, 27, 240–41, 352
Mizar, 349
Monkey, 248
Monkey Clasps Knees, 218
Monkey Dancing, 293, *293*
Monkey posture, 233, *233*
Monkey Prays with Elbows, 218–19,
    218
Monkey Rotates Spine to Leg, *223*
Mountain Rises from the Sea, 220,
    220
Mung Bean Hitting, 257, *257*
muscle cramps, 292–93, *292–93*
Mystic Subtlety, 349

navel, 156–59, *156*, *158–59*
navel, collecting energy in, 19, *19*
neck, 192–93, 240
negative emotions, 3, 4, 9
nerves, 163, 296–98, 338–39
Ninth Wind, 295
North Corner, Left-Hand Form,
    113–20, *114–15*, *117–19*
North Corner, Right-Hand Form,
    124–29, *124–29*
North Pole, 349
North Star, 282, 332
Nose, 35
nothingness, 282
numbness, 296

olfactory glands, 349

Opening and Releasing the Uterus, 360, *360*

Opening the Belt Channels, 196–98, *196*

Opening the Bones, Sacrum, and Governing Vessel, 28–29, *28–29*

Opening the Bridge Channels, 144–46, *145*

Opening the Door of Life, 240–41, *241*

Opening the Functional Channel, 147–49, *147–48*

Opening the Great Bridge and Regulator Channels, 258–61, *258–61*

Opening the Joints, 236–37, *237*

Opening the Lower Tan Tien, 27–28

Opening the Microcosmic Orbit, 30–33, *31–33*

Opening the Middle Tan Tien, 27

Opening the Regulator Channels, 144–46, *145*

Opening the Spinal Joints, 238, *238*

Opening the Thrusting Channels, 190–95, *191*, *195*

Opening the Upper Tan Tien, 26–27, *26*

Opening the Wind Gates, 156–57, *156*, 284–85, *285*

Orgasmic Upward Draw, 62–64, *62*, *64*

orgasms, 333

Ovarian Breathing, 58–60, *59*

Ovarian Compression, 60–61, *61*

ovaries, 174, 362–63, *362*

packing process, 46–49

pain, 296

pakuas, 98–99, *98*, 182–86, *182*, *185*

pancreas, 39, 167

Partner Practice, 254–56, *254–55*

patting, 160

Peacock Looks at Its Tail, 223, *223*

Pearl, 98–99, *98*, 107–9, *108*

penis, 364

Pericardium meridian, 170, 286–87, 344, *344*

perineum, 365

Phecda, 349

pineal gland, 349

Pisces, 247–48

pituitary gland, 349

positive energy, 9

Prime Elixir, 349

Prosperity Storage, 349

prostate, 175, *175*, 365, 367

psoas muscle, 178, *178*

Pull Bow and Shoot the Arrow, 225, *225*

Pull the Silk and Swing the Leg, 311–12, *312*

pulses, 173, 346

Pure Person, 349

purple light, 349

Push/Pull Master Practice, 24–25

Push Strike, 320

quasars, *282*

Rabbit, 248

Rabbit in the Moon, 333

Rabbit posture, 230, *230*

Rainbow Chi, 22

Ram, 248

Rat, 248

Rattan Stick Hitting, 78

Raven in the Sun, 333

Reaching to Heaven, 120

red, 332

red light, 349

red pheasant, 352

Regulator Channels, 144–46, *145*, 258–61, *258–61*

Releasing and Balancing the Anococcygeal Region, 369–70, *369*

Releasing Blood Supply to the Testicles and Penis, 365, *365*

Releasing Sedimentation in the Scrotal Sac, 365

Releasing the Fallopian Tubes, 360, *360*

Releasing the Inner Thigh, *368*

Releasing the Ovaries, 361, *361*

Releasing the Urogenital Diaphragm, 361–62, *361*

Releasing Toxins from the Lymph System, 171–73, *171–72*

Reunion of Heaven and Earth, 4

Rhinoceros posture, 234, *234*

ring muscles, 221–22, *221–22*

River Flows into the Valley, 217

rocking, 160

Rollback, 320

Rooster, 248

sacrum, 28–29, 35, 236, 369

Sagittarius, 247–48

saline, 244

Saturn, 352

sciatic nerve, 176–77, *177*, 370

scooping, 160

Scorpio, 247–48

Scrotal Compression, 85

scrotal sac, 365–66

Sealing the Aura, 266–67, *267*

Second Corner, West (Left-Hand Form), 322–24, *323–24*

Second Healing Sound, 41

Second Level

　Bone Marrow Nei Kung, 70–71, 73–97, *74, 77, 81, 89, 91, 93, 95, 97*

　Fusion of the Five Elements, 71–72, 98–112, *98, 100, 104, 107, 111*

　Inner Structure of Tai Chi, 72, 113–31, *114–15, 117–19, 121–29, 131*

Second Wind, 287

Self-Intercourse, 347

Seventh Wind, 294, *294*

Sexual Chi Kung, 4

sexual energy, 329

　Female Sexual Energy Massage, 91–93, *91, 93*

　Male Sexual Energy Massage, 88–90, *89*

　recycling, 9

　See also Alchemy of Sexual Energy; Healing Love Through the Tao; Taoist Soul Body

Sexual Palace, 358, *358*

Sexual Power Lock Practice (male), 86–87, *86*

shaking, 160

Shaking the Head and Wagging the Tail, *310*, 311

shoulders, 240

Simple Chi Kung, 210–11, 236–41, *237–39, 241*

Single-Hand Push, 120

Single Whip, 320

Six Directions, 24–25, *25*

Six Healing Sounds, 40–45, *40, 42, 45*

explanation of, 10–11

Sixth Healing Sound, 44–45, *45*

Sixth Level, 5, 329–30

Karsai Ne Tsang, 354–72, *354, 356–64, 366–71*

Tai Chi Wu Style, 330–31

Taoist Soul Body, 328–29, 332–53, *332, 335–46, 353*

Sixth Wind, 292–93, *292–93*

skin, 160

small intestine, 162–63, 342

Small Intestine meridian, 342, *342*

Snake, 248

Snake Turns at Wing Point, 221

Solar Bathing, 246, *246*

solar fire, 349

soul body. *See* Taoist Soul Body

Sphincter Ring Muscles, 221–22, *221–22*

Spinal Cord Breathing, 20, *20*

Spinal Cord Microcosmic Orbit, 263

spine, 338–39

spiraling, 160

Spirit Body, 200–201, *201*

spleen, 39, 166, *166*, 341

Spleen Exercise, 44, *45*

Spleen meridian, 341, *341*

Spreading the Energy, 363, *363*

Steaming

Endocrine Glands, 337, *337*

Five Organs, 336, *336*

Spine, Lymphatic System, and Nerves, 338–39, *338–39*

Twelve Organ Meridians, 340–45, *340–45*

stomach, 39, 341

Stomach meridian, 341, *341*

Strengthening Energy Fields, 277–78

Strengthening the Organs and Balancing the Emotions, 275–77, *276*

Stretching the Neck and Shoulders, 240

strong containers, cultivating, 9

Sun, 184, 186

Swallow posture, 232, *232*

Swallow the Saliva, 142

Tai Chi Chi Kung, 72

Tai Chi Fa Jin, 272–73

Completion, 326–27, *327*

First Corner, South (Left-Hand Form), 320–21, *320–21*

North, East, and South Corners (Left-Hand Form), 325

Opening Movements, 319, *319*

Second Corner, West (Left-Hand Form), 322–24, *323–24*

Transition to Right-Hand Form, 325–26, *325*

Tai Chi Wu Style, 330–31
  Eight-Direction Short Wu Form,
    383–84, *383–84*
  Three-Direction Short Wu Form,
    373–82, *373–82*
tangles, 163
Tan Tien Chi Kung, 209–10
  Animal Postures, 230–35, *230–35*
  Empty Force Breath, 227–28, *227*
  Empty Force Exercises, 228–29,
    229
  Warm-ups, 229
Tao, 6–7
Taoist Astral Healing, 270–71
  Balancing the Planetary and Stellar
    Influences, 280–81, *280*
  Balancing Yin/Yang Extremes in the
    Star World, 281–82, *282*
  Connecting to the Stellar and
    Galactic Forces, 278–79, *279*
  Earth-Sun-Moon Triangle, 274–75,
    274
  Strengthening Energy Fields,
    277–78
  Strengthening the Organs and
    Balancing the Emotions, 275–77,
    276
  Yin Stage Awareness, 283, *283*
Taoist Cosmic Healing, 132–33
  Buddha Palm Closing Practices,
    140–42, *141*
  Buddha Palm Opening Practices,
    136–39, *137–38*
  Grasping the Moon, 143–44, *143*
  Opening the Bridge and Regulator
    Channels, 144–46, *145*
  Opening the Functional Channel,
    147–49, *147–48*
  Yin and Yang Channels, 149–51, *150*
Taoist Soul Body, 328–29
  Animal Protection Practice, 352–53,
    353
  Completing, 346–48, *346, 348*
  Connecting with the Big Dipper,
    347–48, *348*
  Coupling, 334–36, *335*
  Kan, 332–33, *332*
  Li, *332*, 333
  Steaming the Endocrine Glands,
    337, *337*
  Steaming the Five Organs, 336,
    336
  Steaming the Spine, Lymphatic
    System, and Nerves, 338–39,
    338–39
  Steaming the Twelve Organ
    Meridians, 340–45, *340–45*
Tao Yin, 209, 215–22
Taurus, 247–48
temples, 349
Tendon Nei Kung, 212–13
  Coordinate with Your Heartbeat,
    250
  Eight Hand and Arm Positions,
    250–53, *250–53*
  Mung Bean Hitting, 257, *257*
  Partner Practice, 254–56, *254–55*
  Structure, Pressure, Tendon Power,
    249–50, *249*
  Wall Practice, 256
tension headaches, 176
Tenth Wind, 296

Testicle Breathing, 83–85, *84*
Testicle Palm Rub, 366–67, *367*
testicles, 364, 366–67
thalamus gland, 349
third eye point, 349
Third Healing Sound, 42–43, *42*
Third Level
  Chi Nei Tsang, *177–79, 181*
  Cosmic Fusion, 133–34, 182–201,
    182, 185, 187, 189, 191, 195–96,
    199, 201
  Healing Energy of Shared
    Consciousness, 134–35, 202–7,
    202, 204–6
  Taoist Cosmic Healing, 132–33,
    136–51, *137–38, 141, 143–45,*
    147–48, 150
Third Wind, 288–89, *288*
Three-Direction Short Wu Form,
  373–82, *373–82*
Three Fires, 24–25, *25*
Three Minds into One, 136
Thrusting Channels, 190–95, *191,*
  195
thymus, 39
Tiger, 248
Tiger Out of the Cage, 315–16, *315*
tongue, 287
transforming chi, 4
Transforming Emotions, 104–5, *104*
Tree Chi Kung, 179–81, *179, 181*
Triple Warmer Exercise, 44–45, *45*
Triple Warmer meridian, 344, *344*
True Lead, 332, 333
True Mercury, 333
Tui, 183, 186

Turning the Wheel, 347–48, *348*
Twelfth Wind, 298
Twelve Organ Meridians, 340–45,
  340–45
Twist Body Like a Snake, 219

Universal Healing Tao, 387–88
  levels of, 5
  system of, 2–5, *6–7*
universal pakua, 185–86, *185*
Upper Tan Tien, 26–27, *26*
Upper Yang Routes, 261
Urinary Bladder meridian, 343, *343*
urogenital diaphragm, 361–62, *361*
uterus, 174, 360, 362, *362*

vagina, 64–65
Valley Orgasm, 67–68, *68*
varicose veins, 301
vena cava, 289–90
Venting Hot Sick Energy, 155, *155*
Venus, 352
Virgo, 247–48
Virtues, 187–89
Virtuous Mind Power, 205–7, *205–6*

waist loosening, 236
Wai T'o Offering the Rod, 305, *305*
Wall Practice, 256
Water, 212
Water Buffalo Emerging from Water,
  52–53, *52*
Wei, William U., 386
weight lifting
  Female Chi Weight Lifting, 96–97, *97*
  Male Chi Weight Lifting, 94–95, *95*

white tiger, 332

Wind Gates, 156–57, *156*

Windmill Exercise, 238, *238*

Wire Rod Hitting, 73–78, *74, 77*

Wisdom Chi Kung, 11–12, 20–23, *20–23*

Wood, 212

World Link of Protection, 134–35, 203–4, *204*

Wu Chi, 282

Yang Position, 50–51, *50,* 52–53

Yang Route, 260–61

yellow phoenix, 352

Yin and Yang Channels, 149–51, *150*

Yin Essence, 349

Yin Position, 50–51, *50,* 53

Yin Route, 258–60

Yin Stage Awareness, 283, *283*

BOOKS OF RELATED INTEREST

Healing Light of the Tao
Foundational Practices to Awaken Chi Energy
by Mantak Chia

Healing Love through the Tao
Cultivating Female Sexual Energy
by Mantak Chia

Chi Self-Massage
The Taoist Way of Rejuvenation
by Mantak Chia

Simple Chi Kung
Exercises for Awakening the Life-Force Energy
by Mantak Chia and Lee Holden

Sexual Reflexology
Activating the Taoist Points of Love
by Mantak Chia and William U. Wei

Cosmic Nutrition
The Taoist Approach to Health and Longevity
by Mantak Chia and William U. Wei

Iron Shirt Chi Kung
by Mantak Chia

Cosmic Detox
A Taoist Approach to Internal Cleansing
by Mantak Chia and William U. Wei

INNER TRADITIONS • BEAR & COMPANY
P.O. Box 388
Rochester, VT 05767
1-800-246-8648
www.InnerTraditions.com

Or contact your local bookseller

31901052027697